And if you think about it, this is the traditional come-on used since Charles Atlas sold courses with the lure that even if you were a 97-pound weakling who got sand kicked in his face now, you could build yourself into something that far transcended your present state. But unlike Atlas's goal of worldly empowerment, the transcendence that Kim is focusing on is a completely internal thing, a process of self-discovery and self-improvement the likes of which nothing else can rival.

The next time you approach the squat bar for yet another set of this most easy-to-hate lift, remind yourself not that this set will bring you one step closer to being like Arnold, but rather that it will bring you one step closer to being what you are and what you can be.

Do it for yourself and the glory of God—there's no better reason, no more powerful motivator, no more rewarding challenge.

As ever, train wisely.

Randall J. Strossen, Ph.D.
Publisher & Editor-in-chief
Nevada City, California

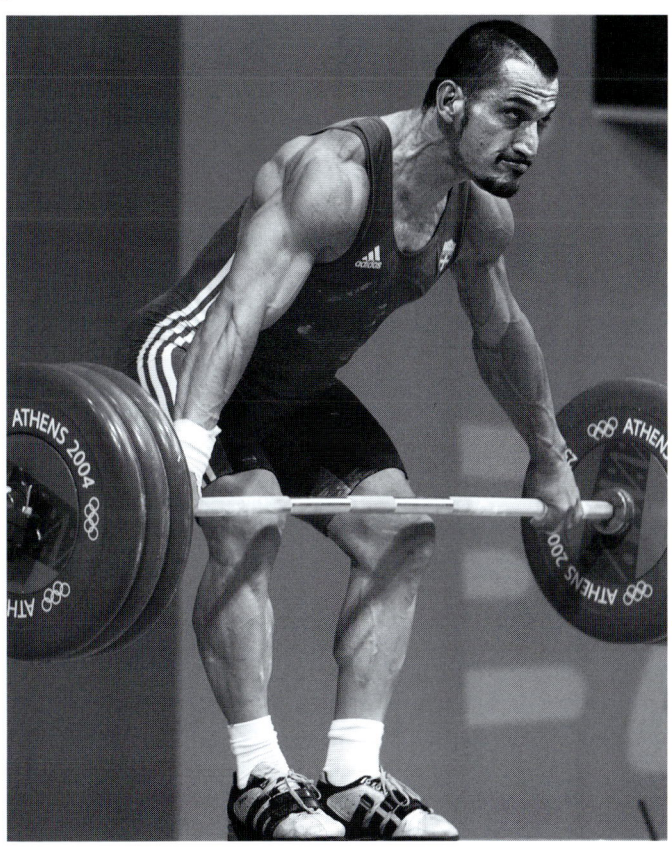

**Pyrros Dimas won three Olympic gold medals in weightlifting and was probably the most financially successful weightlifter in recent time as well. Not everyone can achieve Dimas's competitive or financial success, but the inherent benefits of the sport are available to all.**
Randall J. Strossen photo.

# What For?

One of the hot topics on the IronMind Forum (www.ironmind-forum.com) is a thread called "The Future of Strongman," started by Paul Ohl.

As you would guess, there has been a lot of talk about whether strongman events should be standardized, how strongman could be developed to a level far beyond its current state, the role of drug testing, and so forth. Something of a lone voice in the wilderness has been Kim Wood, as he's emphasized the importance of training for oneself, rather than for others.

But let's back up a minute. If you've never met Kim, this is how I introduced him on the IronMind Forum:

"I noticed that Kim Wood posted on the 'CoC and the NFL' thread today. I wanted to welcome Kim and mention that his background includes three decades as a strength coach for the Bengals. He cut his teeth at Nautilus and helped found, develop and sell HammerStrength, and while it sometimes takes some coaxing to get Kim to speak his mind, I am hopeful we won't feel that the cat got his tongue.

"Incidentally, Kim has long been a quiet benefactor of fledgling companies in the industry. In IronMind's earliest days, his regular orders for a few of this and a few of that put some wind in our sails, and I know he has done likewise with others."

Kim Wood, if you've never met him, is not exactly a shy guy, and he is not afraid to rock the boat or mess with people just because he can. In his student days at the University of Wisconsin, for example, Kim used to warm up at home and then run down to the YMCA, throw 300 pounds on the bar and press it overhead, drawing some looks of amazement as he headed back out the door as suddenly as he appeared.

Drugs in sports is one of Kim's favorite targets, so on this thread, he wasted no time attacking the topic in the spirit of Carrie Nation, but the real axe Kim dropped was much less predictable: he championed training for its own sake, as a means of personal exploration and self enrichment.

Forget the screaming fans, the hordes you wished adored you, says Kim, and focus on what training does for you: enriching your life as it transforms you. Otherwise, you'll likely be distracted, end up disappointed, and almost certainly miss the biggest benefit you could have gotten from your training.

Transformation—physical, mental, spiritual—it's all there as the result of lifting weights. It's something you can't buy, and it's something you are less likely to achieve if you train robotically rather than with individual premeditation . . . but it's the big carrot waiting for you each time you approach a barbell.

# Table of Contents

## Departments

| | |
|---|---|
| 2 | **What For?** by Randall J. Strossen, Ph.D. |
| 4 | **Letters to the Editor** |
| 6 | **From the Trenches: Suburban Strength Assault Mission** by William L. Crawford, M.D. |
| 70 | **Iron Filings** |
| 77 | **Captains of Crush® Grippers: Who's New** |
| 79 | **Calendar** |
| 127 | **The Iron Mine** |

## People

| | |
|---|---|
| 53 | **John Godina: World-Class Throwing Drug-Free** by Thom Van Vleck |
| 114 | **Pudzianowski or Savickas: Who is the Greatest All-time Strongman?** by M. Andrew Holowchak, Ph.D. |

## Training

| | |
|---|---|
| 8 | **Combine and Conquer** by Ken Best |
| 26 | **Pre-Tension for Power** by Pavel |
| 28 | **The Best Workout Ever!** by Steve Jeck |
| 31 | **The Other Modern-Day Epidemic: Stress** by William L. Crawford, M.D. |
| 36 | **Foundations: Controlled Striking for Physical and Mental Toughness** by Jon Bruney |
| 38 | **It's Never Too Late** by Jim Schmitz |
| 48 | **The Primordial Rust Belt Workout: Chained to Power** by Steven Helmicki |
| 50 | **Getting Things Straight, Part II: Hardball Training** by Dr. Ken E. Leistner |
| 58 | **Carnivores and Cancer: Where's the Beef?** by Steve Milloy |
| 62 | **The Country Mile** by John Brookfield |
| 65 | **Running for His Life** by Keith Wassung |
| 68 | **Medicine Ball Throws to Increase Power and Quickness** by Col. (Ret.) Joseph H. Wolfenberger |
| 80 | **How to Live a Lot in One Day** by Myles Wetzel |
| 83 | **Those Awesome Antioxidants** by Bill Starr |
| 92 | **Training for Grip Competitions** by David Hurzeler |
| 102 | **Metabolic Conditioning** by Brian Mangravite |
| 119 | **Philosophy on Strength: What Makes a Person the Strongest?** by Paul Mouser |
| 125 | **Cross Training: Bike Riding** by Steve Justa |

## Contests

| | |
|---|---|
| 12 | **2010 IHGF Heavy Events World Championships: Exciting, Close . . . and Brock Rocked** by Francis Brebner |
| 105 | **2010 dotFit World Strongman Super Series Mohegan Sun Grand Prix: Local Cop Locks Up the Win—Again** by Randall J. Strossen, Ph.D. |
| 123 | **IHGF World Highland Games Series: First Stop, Bressuire, France** by Francis Brebner |

## History

| | |
|---|---|
| 46 | **A Neglected King of Middleweight: Miro Gamba** by Gherardo Bonini |
| 97 | **The Search for Harold Wood** by Roger Davis |

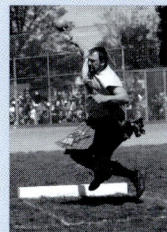

**G-forces on the field of play:** Larry Brock develops some serious rotational inertia on the 28-lb. weight for distance as he spins years of hard work into a big victory at the 2010 IHGF Heavy Events World Championships in Victoria, British Columbia, Canada.
Randall J. Strossen photo.

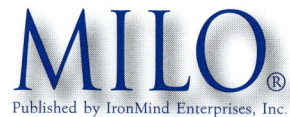

Published by IronMind Enterprises, Inc.

Randall J. Strossen, Ph.D.
*Publisher & Editor-in-chief*

Elizabeth M. Hammond
*Production Editor*

Susan Altman
*Production Assistant*

---

P.O. Box 1228
Nevada City, CA 95959 USA
www.ironmind.com
Tel: +1-530-272-3579
Fax: +1-530-272-3095
E-mail: sales@ironmind.com

MILO is published quarterly:
March, June, September &
December
Subscription rates for
4 books are:
*Softcover:* US$79.95/year USA;
US$89.95/year Canada/Mexico;
US$99.95/year all others
*On-line:*
US$42.95/year all subscribers

Single issues are:
US$20.00 each + $5.00 S&H USA
(US$7.00 S&H Canada/Mexico;
US$13.00 S&H all others)

---

Copyright ©2010
IronMind Enterprises, Inc.

All rights reserved.
No part of this publication
may be reproduced
or transmitted in any form
or by any means without prior
written permission except
in the case of brief quotations
embodied in articles
and reviews.

---

Design:
Tony Agpoon
Sausalito, CA

## Letters to the Editor

### The WOB Made Clear

Just a quick note to say that the article on training and preparing for the weight-over-the-bar event in the Highland Games was outstanding ["Standing Weight-Over-Bar: A Primer Course" by Thom Van Vleck, MILO March 2010, Vol. 17, No. 4]. Can the author be encouraged to back this with a series covering the other staple events that the Highland Games competitors covered? It made the event seem accessible and extremely tempting to have a go at, whereas the Highland Games events seem out of reach and something resembling a black art.

Gareth Shepherd
Pudsey, UK

### Music to Our Ears

Keep up the great work—MILO is certainly the highest quality print journal in the Iron Game today!

John R. Corlett
Davis, CA

### Weightlifting Does It All

*Erőt, Egészséget!* These words are an ancient Hungarian greeting meaning I wish you strength and health! Apparently the ancients were more aware of the value of strength than our contemporaries. Today even the experts are confused and the specialists depend on aerobic magic.

The body is an integrated system: you can't affect one part without influencing others. If you are naturally strong (without drugs), all your body parts will also be strong and you will have what it takes to be healthy. The reverse is also true; I claim only that it is easier to be healthy if you are strong.

In 1952, I participated in a medical test, including a lung capacity test, given by the army sport clubs to their nationally elite athletes. The tests were carried out by army doctors from army hospitals. Soon after testing began, the head doctor announced that the test up to that time had an "unexpected result": the lung capacities of the elite swimmers and the elite weightlifters overlapped. From most of the lung capacity test results, you couldn't tell who were swimmers and who were lifters. This was not unexpected for us lifters, but obviously nobody told the medical authorities that it was a training effect—something they wouldn't know about because it was not common knowledge. So, for instance, when a 90-kg lifter had a larger lung capacity than any swimmer tested up to that time, they quickly dismissed it as an anomaly. This was no anomaly to us—we knew we did not spend time in the gym in vain. We felt great zest for life. Hard workouts were a challenge for us, not a burden. Food and drink were tastier, celebrating and singing was happier, sleep was more restful, and girls' kisses were sweeter.

Olympic-style weightlifting is both a strength and aerobic sport.
    Dezso Ban
    Kunkletown, PA

### Rigert Reaction
The June issue of *MILO* was excellent. I especially liked the photo layout for the Europeans. Rigert is still scary.
    Bill Starr
    Aberdeen, MD

### Got It Straight
Thanks for Dr. Ken's article in the June 2010 *MILO* ["Getting Things Straight, Part I: "Core" Principles"]. The workout is excellent and I'm using it with great results.
    Jeff Vitale
    St. Helens, OR

### *MILO* Guy Encounter
Again, I am blown away by the quality of *MILO*. I got the June 2010 issue today in the mail and just flipping through the authors, topics and pictures, I know this will certainly be a great read. A neurologist friend of mine who had back problems and is now a trap bar as well as *MILO* enthusiast, called me to gush about this month's *MILO* as well. He had been experiencing back problems and had limited time to train. He wanted to get a simple system for total body workouts. I advised him to get a barbell for his body and subscribe to *MILO* for his mind. His back is better and he is hooked on heavy training now. I guess a *MILO* guy lives inside many men's bodies—they only need to come in contact with another *MILO* guy to get on board with the best thing going in strength.
    Bill Crawford, M.D.
    Concord, NH

### More for Dr. Ken
I just finished reading Dr. Ken's article in the March 2010 *MILO* ["A Quick Summary of Strength Training in the Modern Age"]. I am training at Jack King's Gym in Winston [Winston Salem, NC] and when I am done I enjoy reading the mags he has available. Great article on Dr. Ken's take of the strength and conditioning coach. As I begin to work on the private side of things, he is right, and I won't have to worry about the political bull c*** we face when working for organizations.
    Joe Kenn
    Winston, NC

### Correction
It has just come to my attention that I used the wrong name for the Glima organization in my last article ["Glima: Icelandic Folk Wrestling" *MILO*, June 2010, Vol. 18, No. 1]. I referred to the IGF (International Glima Federation) and it should have been the IGA (International Glima Association). People should still be able to get in touch with them through a Google search; the web address is: http://internationalglima.com/.
    Brian Jones, Ph.D.
    Frankfort, KY

## From the Trenches:
# Suburban Strength Assault Mission: Anvils, Stones and Courage
### William L. Crawford, M.D.

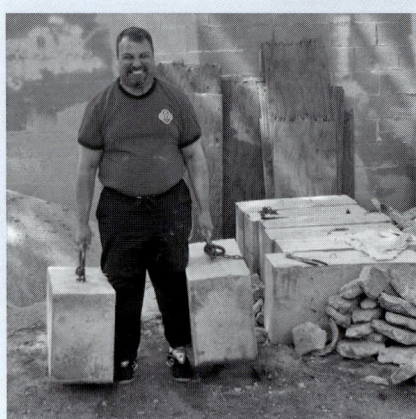

Bill Crawford lifting the concrete blocks (450 lb. each) with no belt and no straps.

Bill Crawford levering a 600-lb. anvil—"a little scary but worth the effort."
Hapy Mayer photos.

May 1 was a day of reckoning for a number of New England strength athletes, including Erik Sauve, Dana Florence, Hapy Mayer, Robert Troupe and me. Robert had arranged for the south shore of Massachusetts to be the site of our challenge with odd and ridiculously heavy implements. Robert advised us to bring camouflage face paint, lifting belts . . . and bail money.

Kidding aside, we started at a local blacksmith shop to lift a 275-lb. anvil from the ground to a 3-ft. stump—this was surprisingly difficult to lift, and now I want my own anvil. This little beast was the warm-up for the whole shindig.

Next we lifted concrete blocks that weighed about 900 lb. combined. Lifting the blocks side to side with the attached steel rings called to mind Jack Shanks's training stones for lifting the Dinnie Stones in 1972 ["Forever Linked: Jack Shanks and the Dinnie Stones" MILO, March 2009, Vol. 16, No. 4]. Standing with 900 lb. is a sobering feat and this was just the start!

We next ventured to a site that had a 24-ft. utility pole that weighed about 800 lb. We worked to shoulder the great piece of wood and collected some splinters along the way. Erik pried a 60-penny nail from the utility pole and bent it several times until it broke.

A trip to a dense thicket alongside a highway was the next destination. Robert had been thinking about tossing a 16-lb. sheaf up to an old billboard for years and now he had ready accomplices. We plowed through the thicket and started tossing a sheaf up at the billboard. Can you imagine the surprise of those on the highway suddenly seeing a bag flying up from the scrub? Robert, a world record holder in the 16-lb. sheaf at 39', banged the sheaf bag several times about 35' up on the billboard, with the rest of us scrambling to find the bag in the brush.

Our last journey was to a heavy equipment garage that housed an ancient anvil—not just any anvil, but a 600-lb. anvil. What the heck were we going to do with that? Housed in a locked garage, we finally got in when Robert found the key the owner kept outside. Robert claimed to have gotten permission to lift the anvil from the owner, but we were beginning to wonder as the local police showed up. Ah, the bail money! Anyway, the owner of the garage, Jack, rolled in just behind the inquisitive policeman to give veracity to the entire situation. We ended up turning the anvil on its end with the

> . . . BUT WE WERE BEGINNING TO WONDER AS THE LOCAL POLICE SHOWED UP.

horn facing up. Levering the beast off the floor a few inches was all that Dana, Erik, Robert, and I could each manage. Bruised and bloodied after this test of fortitude, we heard stories from Jack about the men from the past who had wedged this beast from the ground. We dutifully signed his book of the few who had lifted this great piece of steel from the floor.

To quote Conan, "It is not who won or lost, but that few stood against many." We few men did stand up against very heavy objects and had the time of our lives. Most of us only need to look to ourselves and those few we consider lifting partners to go to extraordinary heights in strength. Organize your own scavenger hunts to complete feats of strength in your area. Anyone have a 600-lb. anvil? M

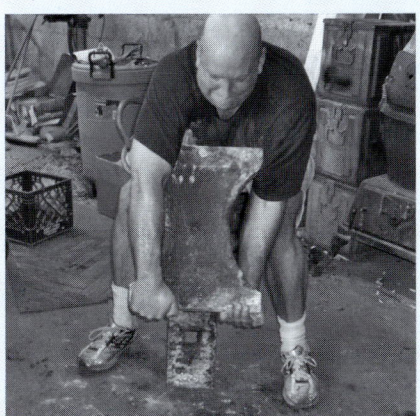

Six-six, 300-lb. Robert Troupe levers the anvil and even he doesn't make the anvil look small!

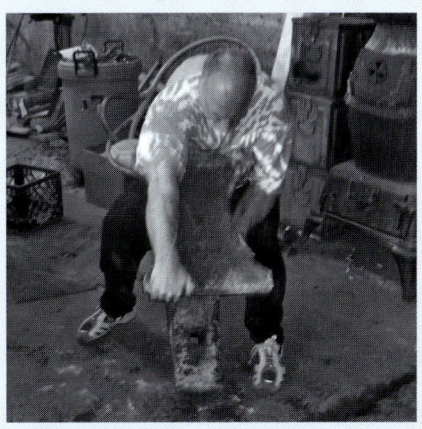

At a bodyweight of 240 lb., Erik Sauve levers the anvil with one hand.
Bill Crawford photos.

# Combine and Conquer
## Ken Best

As I get increasingly busier with a full-time job, writing, and other responsibilities such as helping my wife around the house, raising two school-aged children and caring for my wife's parents (who live with us), I'm finding less and less time to devote to strength training. I've decided that the least amount of strength training I must do to maintain what I've built and to benefit healthwise is exercising twice a week for at least a half hour. I've set a goal that no matter what happens in my life, I'll strive to get those two sessions in without fail.

Fortunately, my full-time job requires a lot of bike riding, so my aerobic training is taken care of. As I get older, it becomes increasingly important for me to pay attention to cardio work in addition to weight work, and my goals have changed somewhat to reflect that. If I have some time on the weekend, I'll do an intense session of skipping or swimming, or talk the family into a swim at the beach or a bush walk in the hinterland to get in some active recovery without it taking me away from other responsibilities. Get the whole family involved, and there's no excuse.

> THE FIRST TIME I SAW WEIGHTLIFTING AT THE 1992 OLYMPICS, I WAS HOOKED. IT REMINDED ME OF MARTIAL ARTS WITH A BARBELL . . .

Up until now, I've stuck to a heavy-light-medium system of training *a la* Bill Starr ["Utilizing the Heavy, Light, and Medium Concept" by Bill Starr, *MILO* September 2009, Vol. 17, No. 2]. When I was laboring all day, I found this system worked well for me because I was often fatigued and injured, and the H–L–M system allowed me to pay attention to rehab exercises on my light day. Now that I spend more time in the office, I have more energy to train, but less time during the week to do so. I can now train only twice a week, so I wanted to make sure I could train hard at each session. This meant consolidating more work into less time.

I'll always be a martial artist at heart, and ever since I lifted my first dumbbell, I tailor my strength training to improve not just strength, but also athletic performance and functional fitness. This is the philosophy that drew me to *MILO* in the first place. It also led me to a brief but successful career as a competitive Olympic-style weightlifter and powerlifter. The first time I saw weightlifting at the 1992 Olympics, I was hooked. It reminded me of martial arts with a barbell, and as soon as I found a place to train, I took to it like a duck to water.

I no longer train in the martial arts; I just don't have the time. But as readers of my previous articles know, I tailor my workouts to mimic the strength and conditioning needed to excel at combat. I like to train multiple muscle groups at once and organize workouts

> WHEN I'M FACED WITH A STRENGTH-TRAINING DILEMMA, MY BRAIN GOES INTO OVERDRIVE TRYING TO RE-ORGANIZE THINGS SO I CAN STILL TRAIN EFFECTIVELY.

into strength circuits to cut downtime to a minimum. But how far could I go? Doing strongman-style training, in which many muscle groups are taxed at once, seemed to be the ideal solution, but after recently moving house, I no longer had the room or equipment to replicate strongman events.

When I'm faced with a strength-training dilemma, my brain goes into overdrive trying to re-organize things so I can still train effectively. I guarantee that the training-related issues you experience are also faced by someone somewhere else in the world. In this case, the first thing I did was some research. Thanks to the Internet, everything I needed was at my fingertips. Everything old is new again, and so it is with strength training. Just when I thought I was beaten, along came a piece of information that showed me all was not lost.

I was surfing the Net one night, and I came across John Wood's website www.oldtimestrongman.com. As I navigated the site, I found pictures and references to the odd feat of heavy supporting. Many professional strongmen, including Goerner, Sandow, Pullum, Brietbart, and Steinborn, dabbled in this feat. Heavy weights provided by large animals, cars, and people were supported in all manner of ways. Some resembled back lifts, hand and thigh lifts, or harness lifts, and others were nothing like the lifts of today. It was a picture of Anton Riha supporting three barbells and a dozen other weights that gave me an idea.

Riha was a Bohemian strongman who in 1890 set a world record for weight supporting whilst standing. He used a special harness rig to hang and support 1,400 lb. on his body. Now I didn't have a special rig, but I did have a hip belt that could serve the same purpose by hanging weights from my hips as I supported or lifted weights with my upper body. By mixing and matching upper- and lower-body exercises, I was able to come up with a short list of combinations I could experiment with to consolidate a lot of lifting into a short amount of time.

> I, LIKE MANY OTHER TRAINEES, HAVE A GLARINGLY OBVIOUS DIFFERENCE IN STRENGTH BETWEEN MY UPPER AND LOWER BODY.

Because of the large difference in strength between my upper and lower body, doing exercises such as dumbbell power cleans and push presses may be great for my shoulders, arms and core but doesn't tax my legs enough to make them stronger. I could pre-exhaust my legs first with hip belt squats or deadlifts, but this takes time I no longer have. What I've done as a result is combine the two exercises—in this case, dumbbell push presses and hip belt squats—into one, so that legs and shoulders both get worked at the same time with the right amount of weight.

I remember reading in *Hardgainer* magazine that Reg Park could squat with 600 lb. and press behind the neck 300 lb. This gave me a benchmark for the percentage of weight I needed to use on both moves so strength was built proportionately between the upper and lower body. Hence, I needed to press half the weight I could squat, but if I held a weight for squats on my shoulders and tried to press it, I'd kill myself. So I put half the weight on my hips and the other half on my shoulders so I could do both exercises at once with the right amount of weight. This system doesn't work for many exercises, but it works for enough exercises for the major muscle groups that you can get two workouts a week out of it for a cycle or two. I've included the ones I've found the best for twice-per-week training. Through trial and error, I successfully combined four exercises into two, and with the right amount of weight and equipment, you can too. The two best exercises are dumbbell shoulder presses with hip belt squats (with a weight pin), and dumbbell shrugs with hip belt squats with a bar.

Hip-belt squats are best done with a barbell so you can get as low as possible without the weights hitting the ground. I like to do them whilst holding a strap or upright so I don't topple over. Now that I planned to press weights at the same time, I found it was safer to attach a weight stack to the hip belt and stand on blocks to squat deeply. With the weights hanging directly under my centre of mass, I felt more balanced to push heavy dumbbells overhead; and because my legs had to be spread apart to allow room for the weight stack, overhead pressing was more practical.

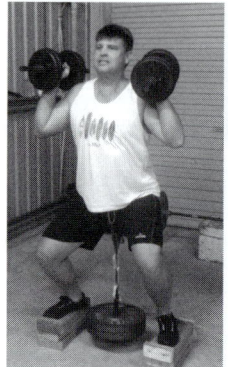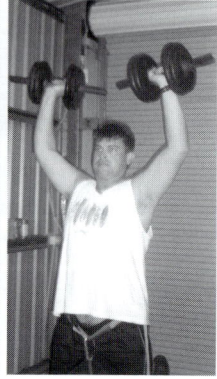

**Squat–press combination.**
All photos by Billy Best.

For the shrug–squat combo, I used a bar with the hip belt and dumbbells for shrugs. The bar allowed me to narrow my stance so the dumbbells, which were held at my sides, didn't bang into my legs with each rep. Also, with the dumbbells held at my sides, balance wasn't a concern, so I could use a bar with the hip belt. You could use a trap bar for shrugs if you have one, as long as you don't lean too far forward during the squat portion; otherwise, you'll crash the bars together and throw off your balance. A trap bar with a weight stack doesn't work unless you have a pile of narrow plates on the stack.

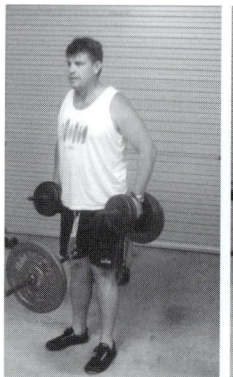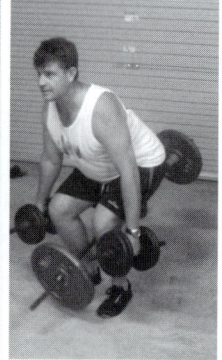

**Squat–shrug combination.**

My workouts now consist of 5 ascending sets of 5 reps on the squat–shrug combo exercise supersetted with weighted ab crunches, and 5 sets of incline dumbbell bench presses supersetted with neck harness work for day one; and 5 sets of 5 reps on the squat–press combo supersetted with side bends, and 5 x 5 on leverage pulldowns supersetted with manual neck work on day two. I add a few sets of squeezes on grippers at the end of each session as a cooldown, and a few quick stretches for hamstrings, quads and shoulders—and I'm done.

Getting into position for these combo lifts is the tricky part. Make sure your area is clear of hazards, such as barbell plates, bars, and slippery surfaces. For the squat–press combo, I set up the weight stack and dumbbells next to a low stool outside of the lifting area. I sit on the stool, attach the belt to the weight stack, bend forward and lift each dumbbell to my knees, and stand up. I wobble over to my blocks, step onto each one carefully, clean the dumbbells to my shoulders and begin the lift. It takes a few reps before I get my balance, but after the first set, I'm in the groove.

For the squat–shrug I do much the same thing, except I'll have the barbell resting lengthways across the stool, sit on it, and attach the hip belt. I lift the dumbbells to my knees as before, stand, walk to the lifting area, and commence. Backing up is a little tricky, but provided I take it slowly, I do okay. If for any reason your flexibility limits your depth in the squatting portion of the lift, work on stretching your calves, hamstrings, and quads. And of course, don't round your back at all during the lifts. It helps to look straight ahead and slightly upward.

I plan on using these combos for three to four months before changing to something else. If time permits, I'll return to a regular routine, but if not, I'll experiment with other combos. Dumbbell deadlifts and a hip belt attached to a bar, combined with stiff-legged deadlifts; and sumo deadlifts with a bar and hip belt attached to a weight stack, combined with bent-over rows are two more moves I could have a go at. And barbell presses (military and behind-the-neck) coupled with hip belt squats with a bar or weight stack are also possible.

Strength training and martial arts share many common philosophies. Setting and achieving goals, overcoming obstacles in life, being physically superior in activities of our choice, and defeating our foes, whether real or perceived, are but a few examples. But where they differ is in how these philosophies are met. In combat and war, particularly where numbers are involved, a tried-and-true method of victory is to divide and conquer. But in strength training when time is of the essence, it seems victory is best achieved when we combine and conquer. Good luck with your training.

> IT TAKES A FEW REPS BEFORE I GET MY BALANCE, BUT AFTER THE FIRST SET, I'M IN THE GROOVE.

# 2010 IHGF Heavy Events World Championships: Exciting, Close... and Brock Rocked

**Francis Brebner**

Seven-time Caber World Champion

Celebrating its 147th year of consecutive Highland Games, Victoria, British Columbia (Canada) was the magnificent setting for this year's IHGF Heavy Events World Championships. Carl Jensen, the athletic director for these Games, along with the Games president Jim Maxwell, went all out to ensure that this championships would be one to remember, and indeed it was. From the moment they arrived in Victoria, it was first-class star treatment all the way for all the IHGF athletes and officials. The host hotel was the Hotel Grand Pacific and grand it was, with its majestic and panoramic views from the hotel suites overlooking the bay and the beautiful city of Victoria. I must say it felt much like Britain.

Jim Maxwell organized a special welcome dinner for the athletes and officials at the Bard & Banker Scottish Pub, where we received a very warm greeting from the Victoria Games committee with a special display of Highland dancing and piping held in our honour.

The lineup of international athletes was twelve in total, three of whom were making their debut: Canadians Jason Johnston and Lyle Barron, and also the much talked-about Polish giant Sebastian Wenta. Wenta has made a great impact on the Scottish Games circuit in the last few years and was tipped to be a possible winner of the championships, but this being his very first Games of the season, the odds were more with favorites Sean Betz and

Larry Brock, who were both on form and showing great marks earlier in the season.

## Day one

On the first day of the championships, you could see the excitement on the faces of the athletes as they were led into the main area by the clans and the mass pipe bands. Thousands of spectators applauded as each athlete was introduced at the opening ceremonies by IHGF president David Webster, OBE; the Games were then officially opened and the championships got under way.

The first event was the 26-lb. Braemar stone, an event that favored England's Scott Rider and Poland's Wenta, both of whom come from a very strong background in track and field with the shot. As for Brock (USA), in past world championships his stone putting had not been as consistent as some of his best events, like the hammer and weight for distance, and had lost him valuable points. But Brock had worked very hard over the winter months and knew all too well that he needed to place at least in the middle of the pack in both stones if he were to have chance of winning the title in Victoria.

Canadian Greg Hadley was first to set his mark with a put of 33' 4"; he was followed by fellow countryman Jason Johnston, who landed a put of 36' 5", ahead of Hadley. USA's Betz opened with 35' 11" and looked very content; as for Brock, all he could muster was a put of 33' 7" and he did not look pleased at all. Next up was a very confident-looking Rider who blasted out a distance of 38' 1", taking the lead; however, this was to be short-lived as Wenta surpassed Rider with a substantial distance of 39' 9-1/2".

In the second round Betz improved slightly, nudging up to 36' 10"; Harrison Bailey III (USA) generated his best of 35' 3", as did Rider with 38' 10-1/2".

In the final round, amazingly both New Zealand's Pat Hellier and Betz matched throws of 36' 10-1/2" for a tie. Wenta also let fly another splendid put, which equaled his first round mark of 39' 9-1/2" for the win. Rider stood firmly in second place with 38' 10-1/2", and Hellier and Betz tied for third place with 36' 10-1/2".

The next event was the 56-lb. weight for distance and it was very exciting to watch as most athletes let loose with throws between 38' and 40'. But for Brock, the world's current number-one ranked weight thrower, this was his specialty and he was confident that he could make up lost ground and earn some valuable points. Brock delivered a throw of 45' 6" in crushing style while letting out his familiar southern trademark yell, "Oh yeah, baby, it's a big one!"

> BUT BROCK... KNEW ALL TOO WELL THAT HE NEEDED TO PLACE AT LEAST IN THE MIDDLE OF THE PACK IN BOTH STONES IF HE WERE TO HAVE CHANCE OF WINNING THE TITLE IN VICTORIA.

> BROCK DELIVERED A THROW OF 45' 6" IN CRUSHING STYLE WHILE LETTING OUT HIS FAMILIAR SOUTHERN TRADEMARK YELL, "OH YEAH, BABY, IT'S A BIG ONE!"

In the second round Betz knew he had to bring his best to the table, and indeed he moved it up a gear as he pulled out a throw of 42' 4". USA's Kerry Overfelt lived up to expectations with his throw of 43' 8-1/2".

In the final round Johnston totally surprised us all with a throw of 43' 2", which moved him into third place over Betz. His lead was momentary as Betz, now in a frenzy, stormed to the trig and let fly with a throw of 43' 7" to pip Johnston by inches and regain his third-place position. Brock went next for his final attempt and with no pressure, lobbed a distance of 44'. He was followed by Wenta, who calmly plopped out a throw of 42' 6", earning himself a fifth-place standing and some valuable points. The top three were: first place, Brock with 45' 6"; second place, Overfelt with 43' 8-1/2"; and third place, Betz with 43' 7".

The 16-lb. hammer was next and the results were very surprising. In the first round most athletes were throwing marks between 115' and 128'—except for Brock, who was looking very calm and confident with one win under his belt and in the mood to add another. He set sail an incredible opening effort of 137' 4" to take the lead by storm.

I could tell by looking at most of the athletes and their form in this event that many were getting tense from nerves, restricting their radius with the hammer and losing feet off their throws—a sure sign of the pressure getting to them.

In the second round Bailey upped his best to 129' 7-3/4". Brock once more established his supremacy with another superb throw of 135'; and Sebastian Wenta improved enormously on his first round throw of only 114' 6" with a second throw of 126' 11-1/2", which left the Polish giant looking well pleased.

In the final round a few athletes showed slight improvement. Betz and Hadley had matching throws of 128' 2"; but it was Scotland's Craig Sinclair who really dug deep and pulled out 131' 6" for second place. Unfortunately for Bailey, Sinclair's result pushed him back into third place with his best throw of 129' 7-3/4", and once again Brock had another win to his credit with a best of 137' 4".

In the caber toss—with a caber 18' 6" long and an incredible 155 lb.—Rider and Wenta shared the first round by both slamming a 12:00 toss. Brock turned out a very good toss at 11:50 and Hadley had a 9:15. With only a 75 degree attempt for Betz, the pressure was on and you could see it written all over his face.

In the second round both Rider and Wenta brought forth the goods again, with Rider outgunning Wenta with a 12:05 toss over Wenta's 12:30. At this point the athletes began to dig deeper and gave their all as they knew not being able to get a score on the caber would dramatically affect the outcome of the championships for them. Next up was Betz, who managed to turn the beast for a 1:45, giving a sigh of relief in the process. Holland's Hans Lolkema followed with a 12:45, Johnston with a 9:45, and Brock with a 2:45.

> NEXT UP WAS BETZ, WHO MANAGED TO TURN THE BEAST FOR A 1:45, GIVING A SIGH OF RELIEF IN THE PROCESS.

The final round showcased perhaps the wrap-up of some of the best caber tossing I have ever seen by Rider, who was successful with an 11:50 score. Combined with his previous tosses of 12:00 and 12:05, these put him ahead of Wenta, who placed second on countback with his three attempts of 11:00, 12:30 and 12:00. In third place was Brock with 11:50, 2:45 and 2:30.

The last event of the first day's championships was the 56-lb. weight over the bar, and with the opening height at 14', all athletes cleared it with no problem. The bar was raised to 15' and Hellier was the only one to make a sudden exit. At 16' Brock, Betz and Wenta cleared it with ease, but unexpectedly Lolkema, Hadley, Overfelt, Sinclair, Johnston, Bailey, Rider and Canada's Lyle Barron all went out at this height.

Wenta and Betz cleared 16' 6", leaving Brock to depart from the competition happy with his third-place finish. With the bar raised to 17' both Betz and Wenta did battle, but neither athlete cleared it so the victory went to Wenta on countback, with Betz in second place and Brock in third.

After the first day, the points were very close between the top four athletes:

| | | |
|---|---|---|
| 1. | Larry Brock and Sebastian Wenta | 17 |
| 3. | Sean Betz and Scott Rider | 19 |
| 5. | Jason Johnston | 28 |
| 6. | Harrison Bailey III | 29 |
| 7. | Craig Sinclair | 38 |
| 8. | Greg Hadley and Kerry Overfelt | 39 |
| 10. | Lyle Barron | 42.5 |
| 11. | Hans Lolkema | 46 |
| 12. | Pat Hellier | 46.5 |

That evening following the competition, all athletes were invited to an all-you-can-eat barbecue hosted by Carl Jensen and his wife; it was much appreciated by the athletes, who afterward turned in early in preparation for the final day of competition the next morning.

## Day two

The athletes were eager to get into the thick of the fray on the second day of competition. After the introduction of the athletes, the competition got underway with the 17-lb. open stone. This event was vital to Brock in the overall standings, and he needed to place at least in the middle of the group.

In the first round Overfelt opened with a put of 39' 5", well below his average. He was followed by Johnston and Hadley, who had puts of just over 45', but it was Hellier who startled some with a 48' 11" result. Rider followed and blasted the stone 51' 3-1/2" to take the lead, which was then flattened by the big man Wenta and his throw of 52' 5".

> RIDER FOLLOWED AND BLASTED THE STONE 51' 3-1/2" TO TAKE THE LEAD, WHICH WAS THEN FLATTENED BY THE BIG MAN WENTA AND HIS THROW OF 52' 5".

Brock's turn was next. As he made his way to the trig, talking to himself and repeating "give just one . . . just one," he began his throw, driving forward and landing in the power position. You would have thought a cannonball was exploding from him as he let rip with his rebel yell, putting the stone a distance of 47' 10", which placed him now in fourth position.

In the second round Pat Hellier upped his mark with a best of 49' 8". The

Flying Dutchman Lolkema was hot on his heels with a fine throw of 48' 5-1/4". Rider then pulled out his best put of the competition with 52' 3", and Wenta once again dominated the event with another marvelous put, this one 54' 9-1/4". Sean Betz made a big impact with a throw of 49', which pulled him well up in the placings.

In the final round, only a few athletes improved their marks, one of them being Lolkema with his put of 48' 7-1/2". Wenta unleashed the biggest throw of 55' for the win. Rider was in second place with 52' 3"; Hellier in third with 49' 8"; Betz in fourth with 49'; Lolkema in fifth with 48' 7-1/2"; and Brock sitting happily in sixth with 47' 10".

With only two more events left, the 28-lb. weight for distance and the 22-lb. hammer, Brock and Betz were the favorites. Brock had placed where he needed to in the open stone and now it was a case of just holding himself together and making no mistakes as the title was within reach.

In the 28-lb. weight for distance, Bailey was first up and heaved a throw of 81' 3-1/4"; Rider was close behind with a throw of 79' 1/4". Next up was a very determined Betz, who walked to the trig and pulled out a class throw of 83' 7". As Brock prepared at the trig, he took a moment to look at where Betz had landed and muttered a few words to himself as he set off in his turns with increasing speed. He planted himself at the finish in great position and ripped out a world-class throw of 89' 1/4". At this point, each athlete knew that it was going to take everything he had to get ahead of Brock.

A few did raise their game: Bailey first with a throw of 84' 1", followed by Rider, who gave his all with a throw of 82' 1", and then Wenta with 80' 5-3/4" and Betz with 83' 8".

In the final round, the improvements were only by inches, with Brock holding steadfast with his spectacular opening throw of 89' 1/4"; Bailey finished in second with 84' 1"; and Betz came in third with 83' 8".

> YOU COULD NOT HAVE WISHED FOR A CLOSER FINISH AND IT ALL CAME DOWN TO THE LAST EVENT.

Going into the last event, the 22-lb. hammer, there was a tie for first place between Brock and Wenta with 24 points each. Rider stood in third place with 25 points and Betz in fourth place with 26 points. You could not have wished for a closer finish and it all came down to the last event.

Sinclair was first up and he whipped out a throw of 110' 11"; following him was Scott Rider with his best of 105' 2-1/2". Sebastian Wenta was having some difficulty finding his form and could only manage a throw of 98' 7", which was a major setback for the Polish giant as this was the event where it mattered most. Hadley produced his best effort of 109' 4", with Betz feverishly following with a sailing throw of 99'. Next up was Brock who looked more determined than I have ever seen him. Once again he went through his ritual of talking to himself, repeating, "Just one . . . give me just one." Brock did just that as his self-belief produced a massive throw of 115' 10", to which Brock said, "That's it, baby!"

In the second round only two athletes improved: Bailey had a fair leap, adding over 5' with a new best of 107'

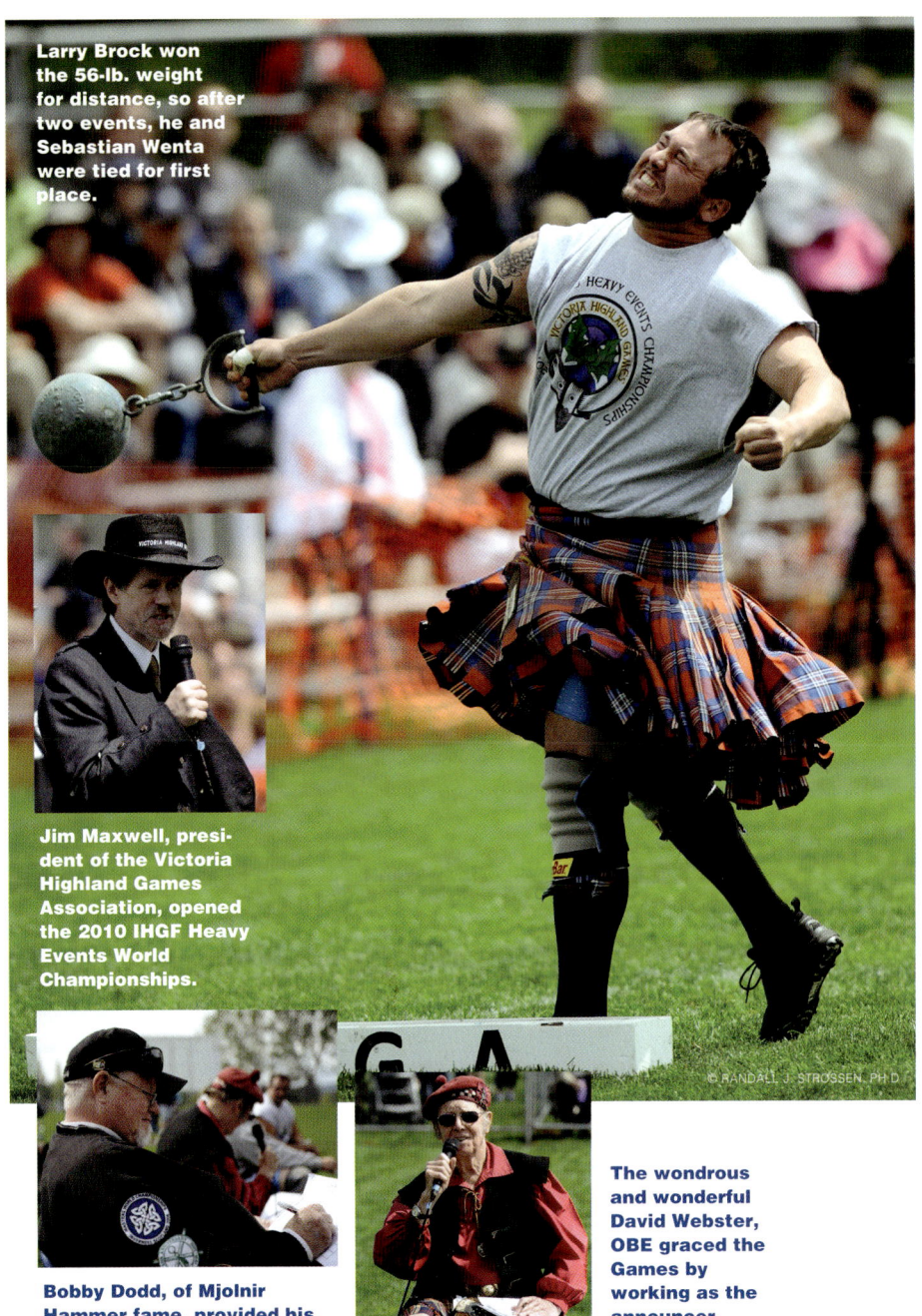

Larry Brock won the 56-lb. weight for distance, so after two events, he and Sebastian Wenta were tied for first place.

Jim Maxwell, president of the Victoria Highland Games Association, opened the 2010 IHGF Heavy Events World Championships.

Bobby Dodd, of Mjolnir Hammer fame, provided his services as a scorekeeper along with his signature hammers.

The wondrous and wonderful David Webster, OBE graced the Games by working as the announcer.

All photos by Randall J. Strossen.

MILO | September 2010, Vol. 18, No. 2   **17**

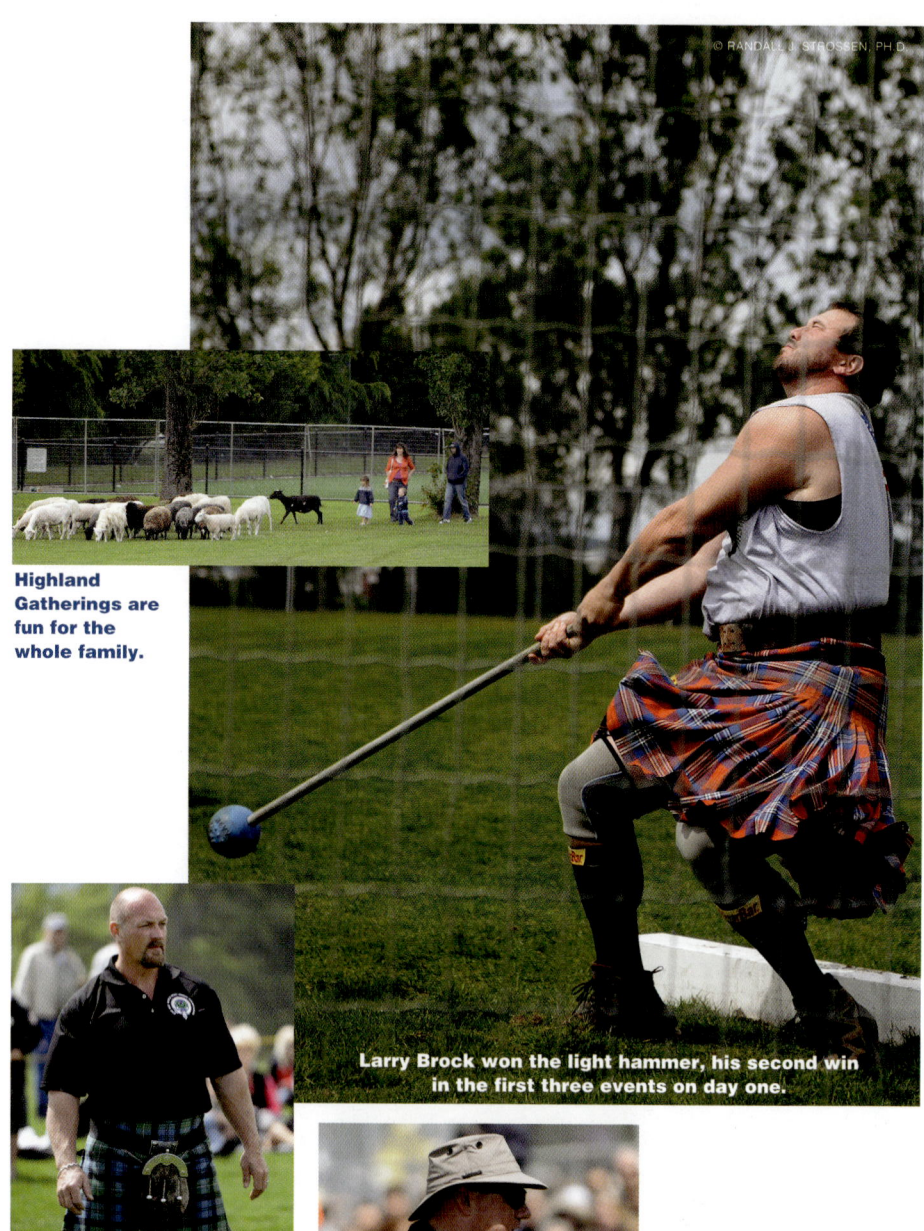

Highland Gatherings are fun for the whole family.

Larry Brock won the light hammer, his second win in the first three events on day one.

IHGF vice president Francis Brebner looks as if he could still do some serious damage as a competitor if he were so inclined.

Carl Jensen, the Games' athletic director, makes an open stone look like a mere egg.

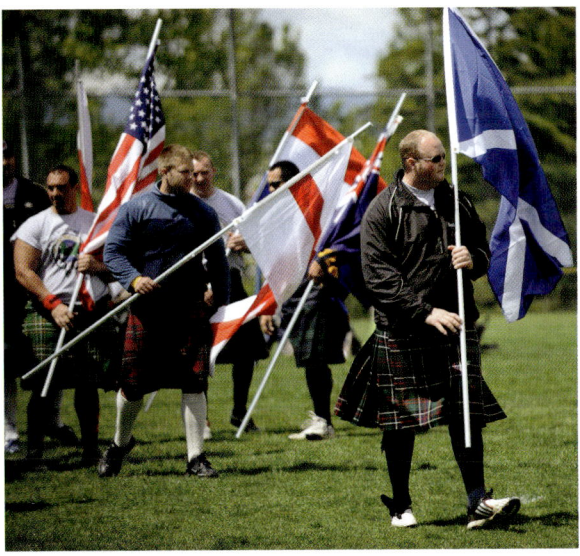

Talk about being cool in the face of pressure: Ray Siochowicz has the vital job of tallying the final scores while athletes, officials, and journalists press for the final decision.

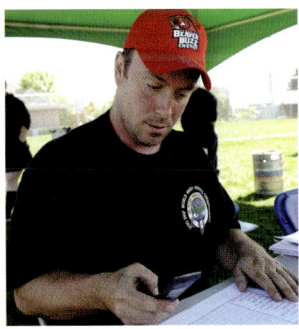

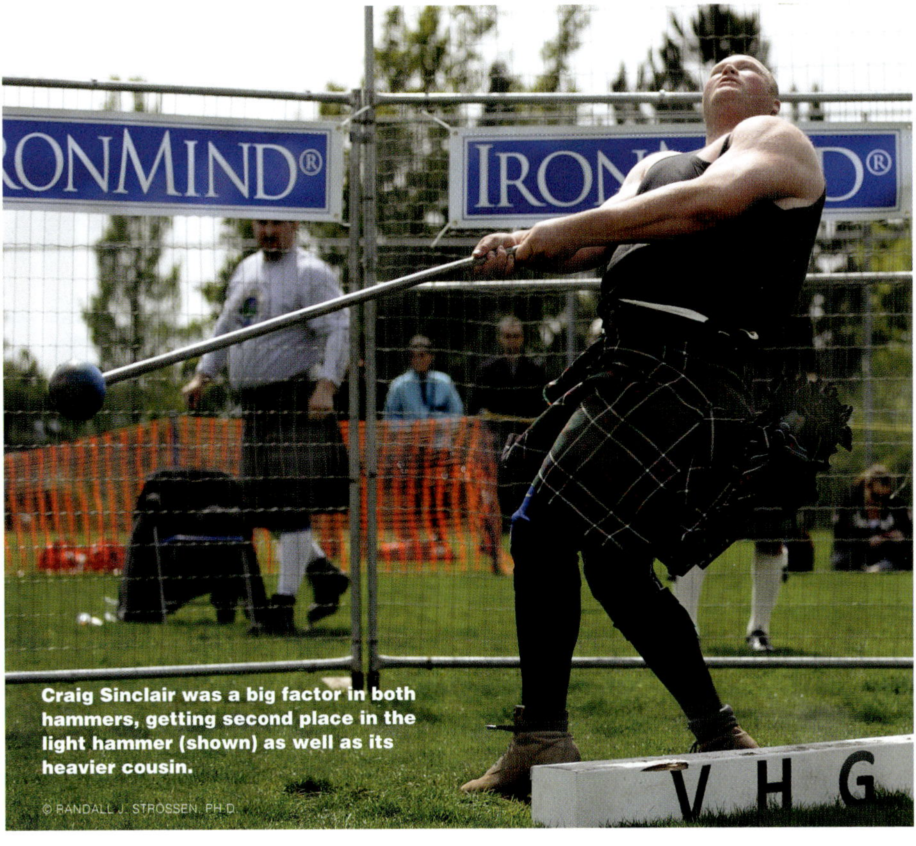

Proudly bearing his country's flag, Scotland's sole competitor, Craig Sinclair, led the athletes' procession.

Craig Sinclair was a big factor in both hammers, getting second place in the light hammer (shown) as well as its heavier cousin.

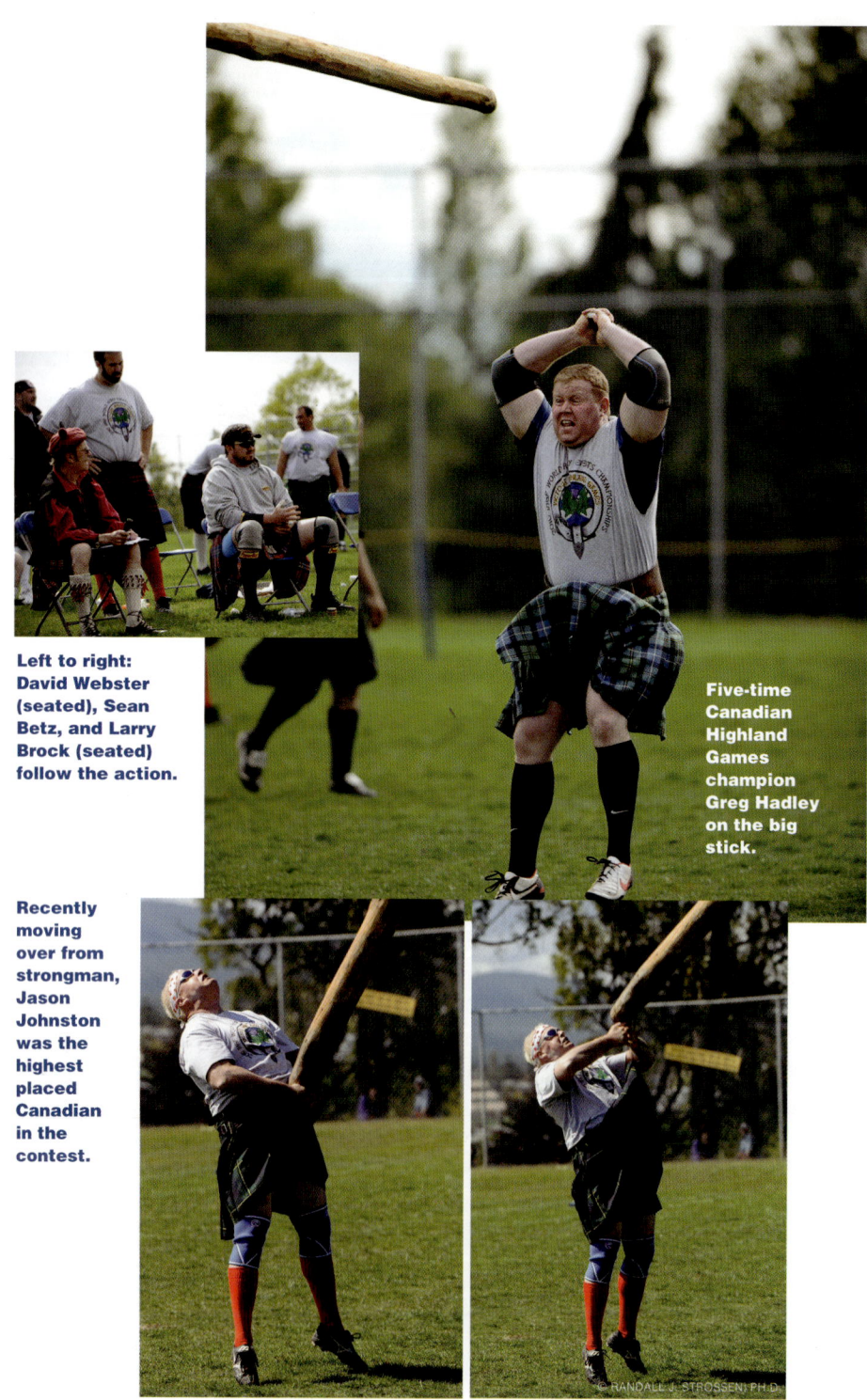

Left to right: David Webster (seated), Sean Betz, and Larry Brock (seated) follow the action.

Five-time Canadian Highland Games champion Greg Hadley on the big stick.

Recently moving over from strongman, Jason Johnston was the highest placed Canadian in the contest.

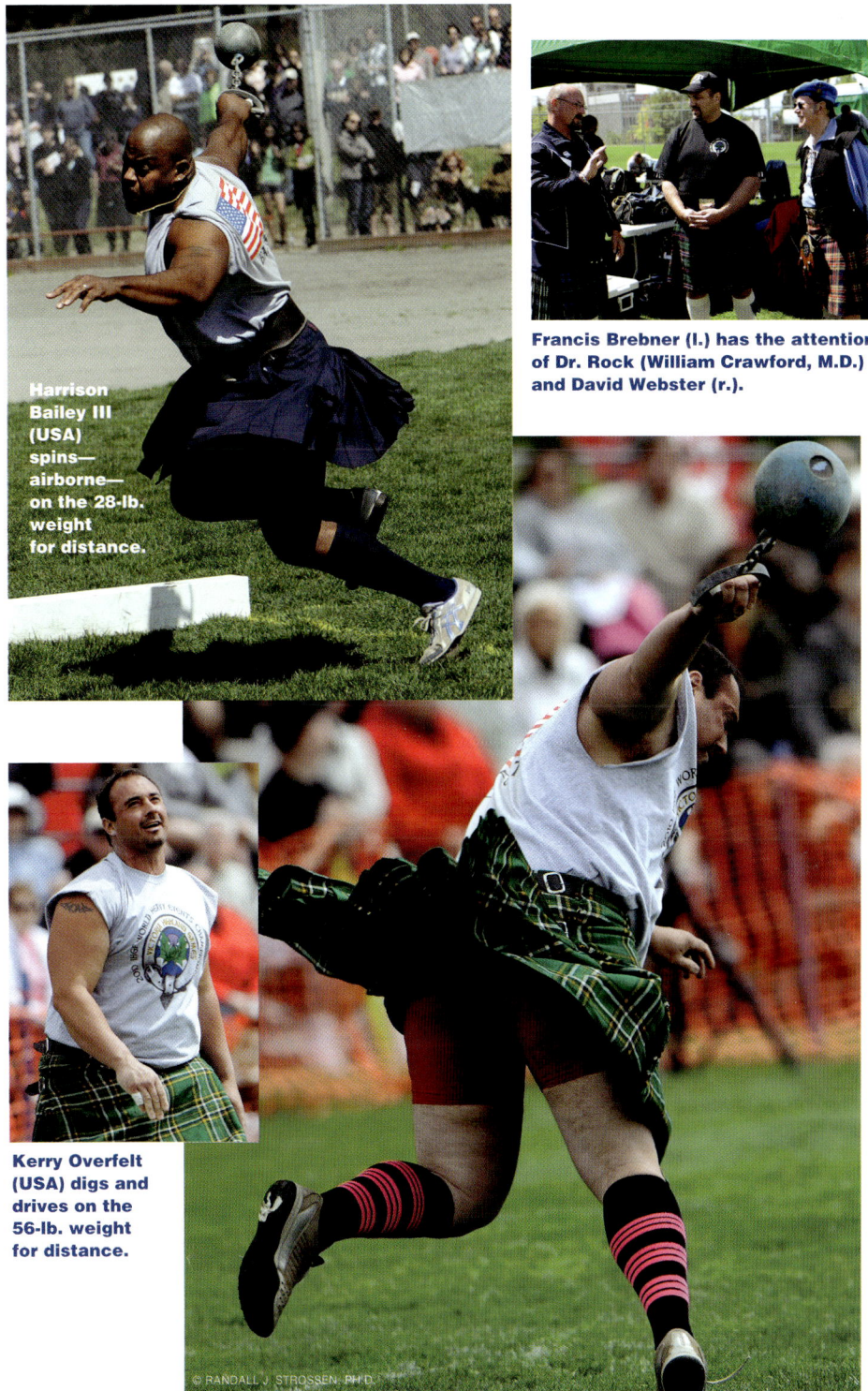

Harrison Bailey III (USA) spins—airborne—on the 28-lb. weight for distance.

Francis Brebner (l.) has the attention of Dr. Rock (William Crawford, M.D.) and David Webster (r.).

Kerry Overfelt (USA) digs and drives on the 56-lb. weight for distance.

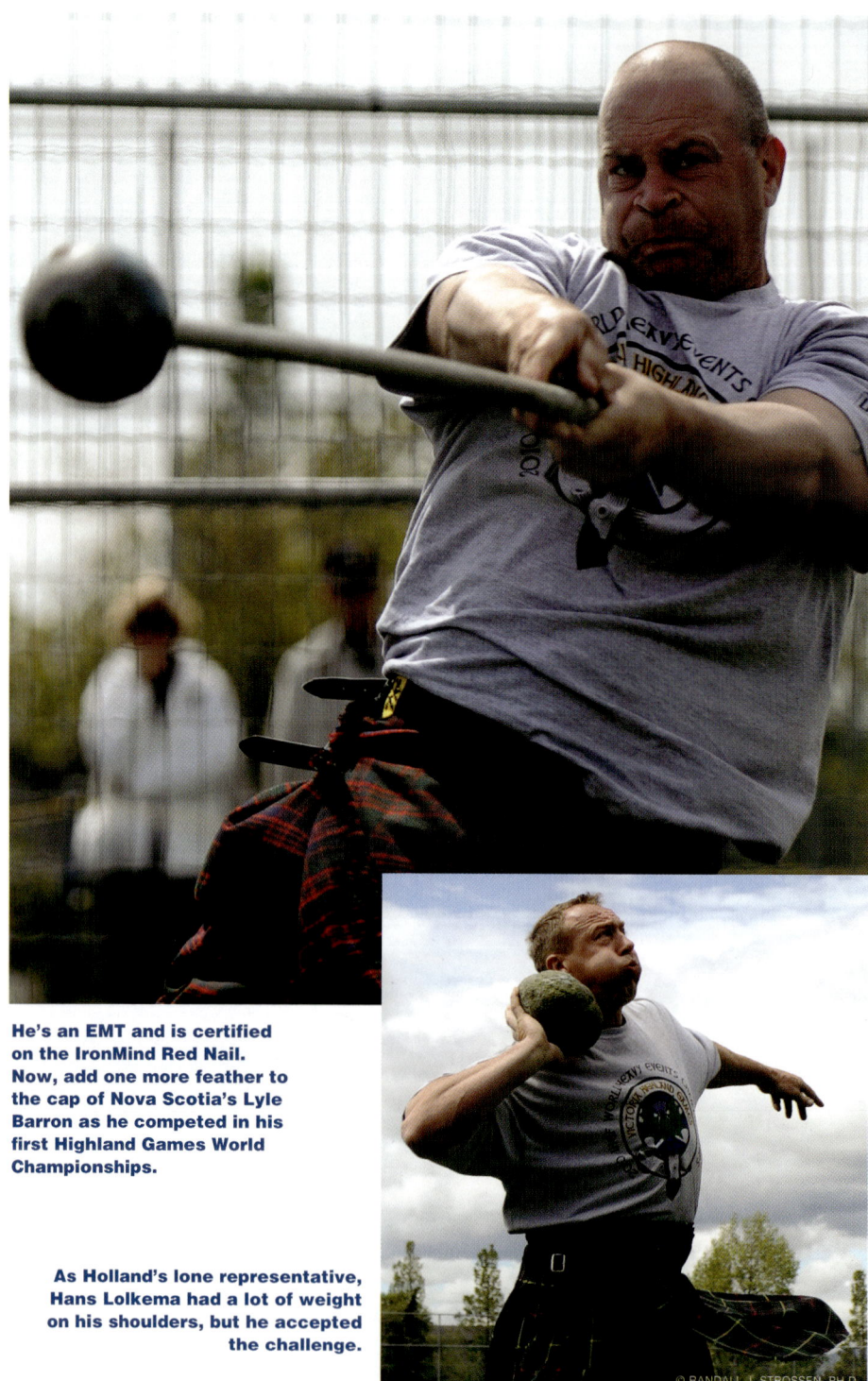

He's an EMT and is certified on the IronMind Red Nail. Now, add one more feather to the cap of Nova Scotia's Lyle Barron as he competed in his first Highland Games World Championships.

As Holland's lone representative, Hans Lolkema had a lot of weight on his shoulders, but he accepted the challenge.

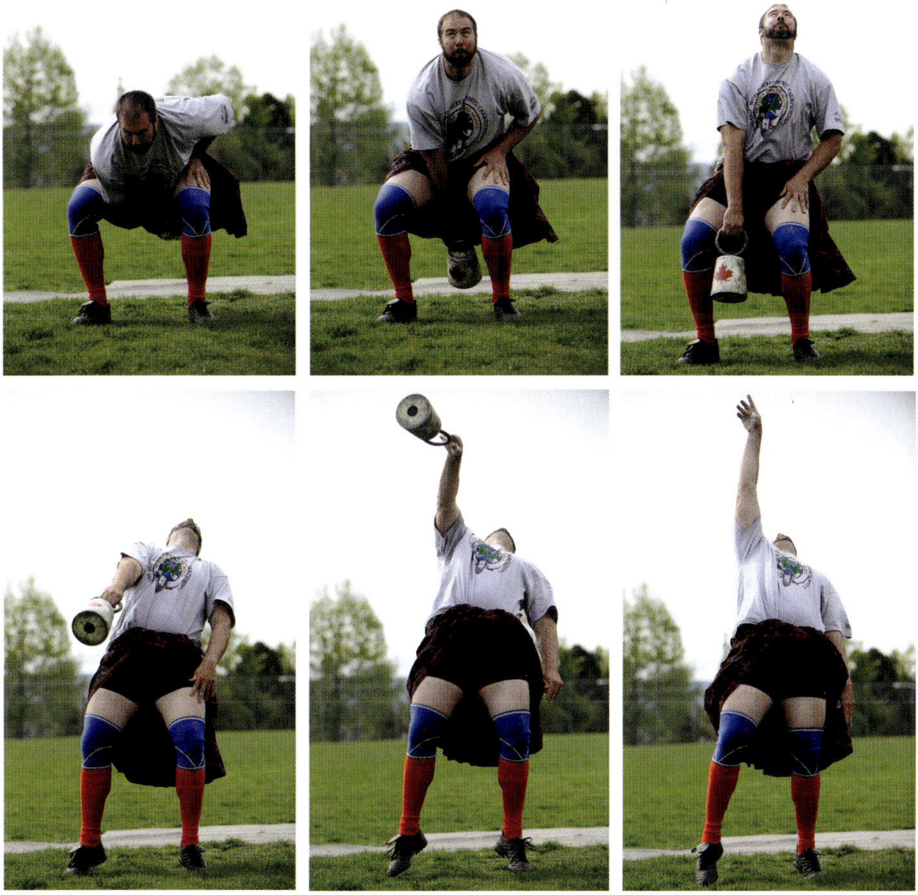

**Sean Betz (USA) bends, swings, extends and explodes, launching the 56-lb. weight for height into space.**

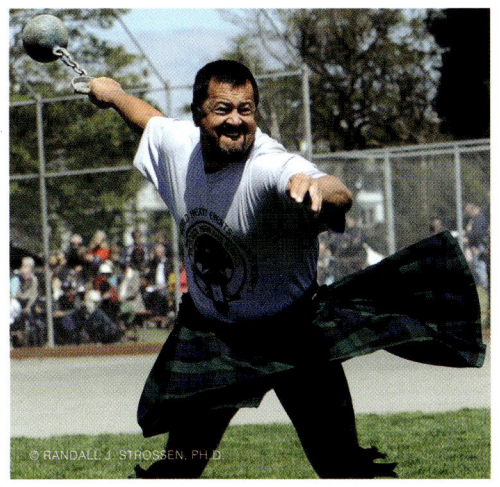

**New Zealand's Pat Hellier is the man with the most Highland Games World Championships appearances under his belt.**

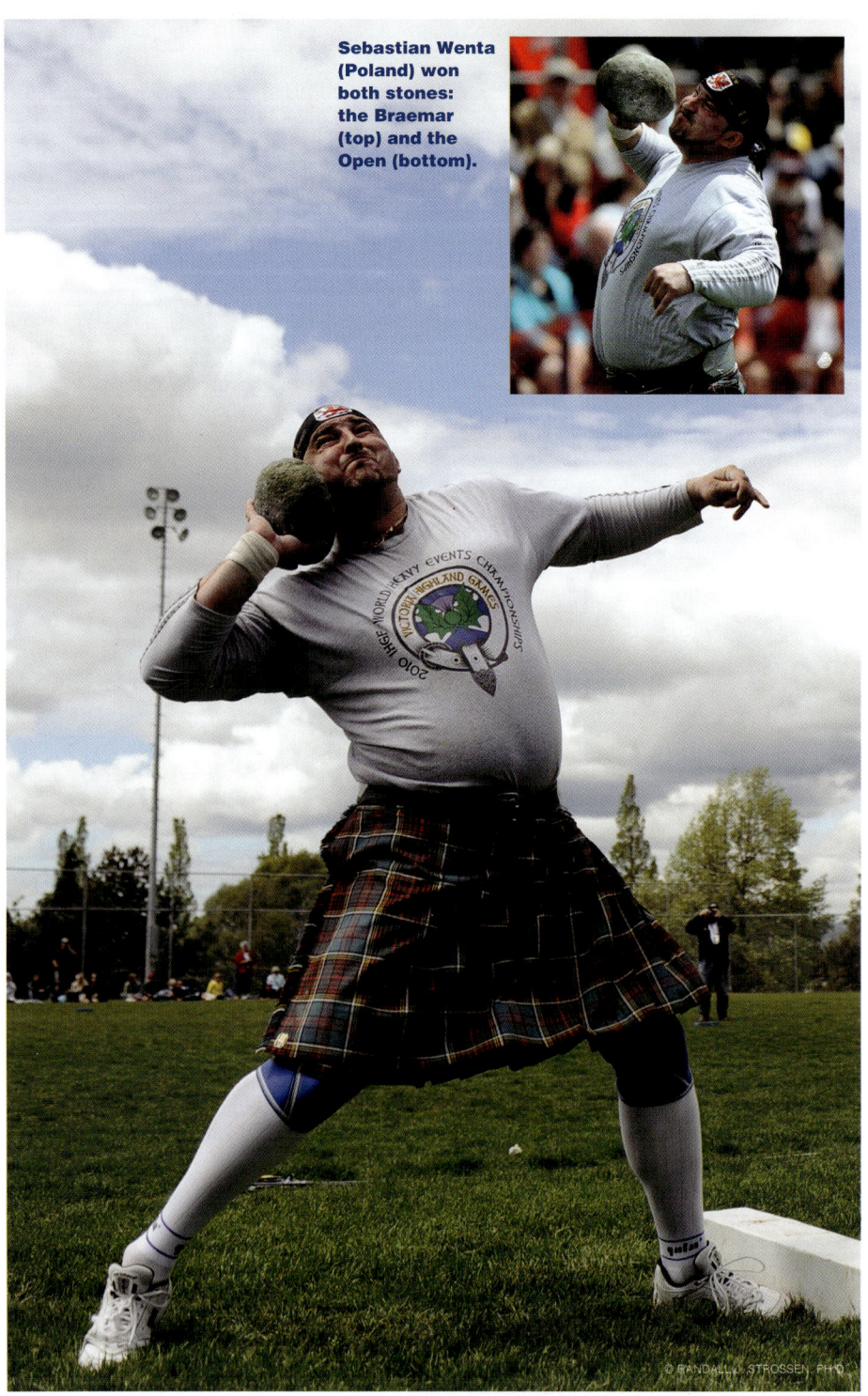

Sebastian Wenta (Poland) won both stones: the Braemar (top) and the Open (bottom).

> GOING INTO THE FINAL ROUND IT WAS CLEAR THAT BROCK HAD ONE HAND ON THE TROPHY, BUT THERE WAS STILL AN OUTSIDE CHANCE THAT WENTA COULD CAUSE AN UPSET . . .

9-1/2", and Betz also added a few feet with a throw of 103' 2-1/2".

Going into the final round it was clear that Brock had one hand on the trophy, but there was still an outside chance that Wenta could cause an upset, as in the past he had thrown over 115' in competition against Brock and beaten him.

Sinclair made his way to the trig and gave his all in his final attempt, improving slightly with a throw of 111' 2". Next came Wenta—for him this was an all-or-nothing throw, but his 103' 4-1/2" fell well short of what he needed to surpass Brock. With his final throw, Betz finished with a best of 108' 2" and in the process moved up four places to fourth. But it was Brock who was the victor, claiming first place with 115' 10"; in second place was Sinclair with 111' 2"; and in third place Hadley with 109' 4".

Brock was this year's winner of the IHGF World Heavy Events Championships, and he had garnered his victory in style by winning the hammer event by several feet and the overall with five clear points.

**Overall Points**

| | | |
|---|---|---|
| 1. | Larry Brock (USA) | 25 |
| 2. | Sean Betz (USA) | 30 |
| 3. | Scott Rider (England) and Sebastian Wenta (Poland) | 32 |
| 5. | Harrison Bailey III (USA) | 45 |
| 6. | Jason Johnston (Canada) | 53 |
| 7. | Craig Sinclair (Scotland) | 58 |
| 8. | Greg Hadley (Canada) | 61 |
| 9. | Kerry Overfelt (USA) | 65 |
| 10. | Pat Hellier (New Zealand) | 70.5 |
| 11. | Hans Lolkema (Holland) | 72 |
| 12. | Lyle Barron (Canada) | 80.5 |

Asking Brock about his titled win, he replied emotionally, "It feels so great to finally win. In the past I have come so close, being runner-up on several occasions. To win the championships in what I consider to be the best lineup of athletes ever at a world championships makes me very happy."

When asked about his preparation for the championships Brock said, "I worked very hard on my weak events, such as my stones, over the winter months and just kept hard at it and it all paid off. I am now looking to have a break for a few weeks before I focus on this year's IHGF World Highland Games series beginning in Bressuire, France, which I am very excited about."

Regarding his performance and second-place finish, Betz said, "I was not at the best I could have been on the day for these championships, but in a field of athletes like this, I am very happy to take second place. As for Larry, he earned it. He came ready on the day and delivered the goods with an exceptional performance all around. I take my hat off to the man: he is a great athlete and true champion and I am happy for him—he deserved it."

Finishing off with a quick word from Rider, asking him about his overall finish, he said, "I am very happy. I managed a few personal bests with the 56' weight for distance and the heavy hammer, I threw at my best, and I am still improving and have my sights set on next year's worlds where hopefully it will be my time to shine."

# Pre-Tension for Power
### Pavel

When I first armwrestled a professional, I got annihilated. Dave Bauer loaded his muscles with maximum tension, to the point of shaking, before we even gripped hands. On the "Go!" he flashed my arm to the table. When he hit me, it was too late for me to load. At 177 lb. soaking wet, this wrist-wrestling world champion dispatched much huskier amateurs than me with casual ease. Bauer's mastery of the skill of getting tight in advance of action played a key part in his winning record.

According to Verkhoshansky (1977), isometrically tensing one's muscles before a dynamic contraction can improve performance by up to 20%. All elite armwrestlers, weightlifters, powerlifters, strongmen, and gymnasts know this. Consciously or not, they are all masters of pre-tension. "I turn myself into a rubber band, I am ready to accept the weight and toss it back up," Ernie Frantz famously said. "If the body is tight it can accept any shock," clarified the powerlifting great, who had instinctively taken the right track in his training and whose book Ernie Frantz's *Ten Commandments of Powerlifting* had the rare honor of being translated into Russian. "If someone were to hit you in the stomach it might hurt, but not if you tensed your stomach muscles first."

In other words, you need to practice maximally tensing your body before you unrack a heavy squat, squeeze off a heavy pull, or perform any other MILO-esque manly effort. All the top guys are already doing it. The following plank-based drills will help you acquire their level of pre-tension skill more quickly.

> ... ISOMETRICALLY TENSING ONE'S MUSCLES BEFORE A DYNAMIC CONTRACTION CAN IMPROVE PERFORMANCE BY UP TO 20%.

The first drill is the full-contact plank. Drop into a regular plank, get tight, breathe shallowly, and ask your training partner to give you some tough love of carefully placed kicks, punches, and shoves against your midsection, armpits, and thighs to stimulate greater tension. I am sure you will not have to ask twice.

Feel free to add an American twist to this Russian standby to make it even more effective. Gray Cook, RKC carefully kicks the soles of the athlete's bare feet with the edge of his foot to stimulate various intrinsic muscles of the midsection.

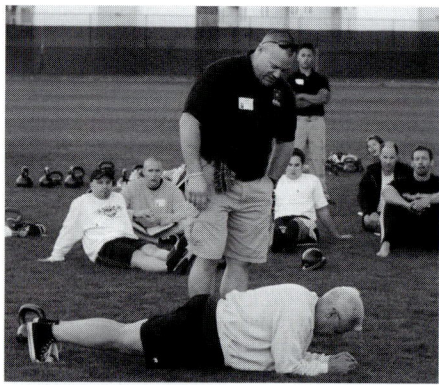

USAPL national champion and IPF Team USA head coach Dr. Michael Hartle, RKC TL giving tough love to masters' IPF world champion Doug Dienelt, RKC.

Photos courtesy www.RKC.com.

The second drill is the drop plank, a favorite of Mark Reifkind, who has a remarkably diverse and rich strength background, including gymnastics, bodybuilding, powerlifting, and kettlebells, not to mention writing a couple of MILO articles. The drop plank goes back to Rif's gymnastics glory days.

Assume the push-up position with your elbows locked. Push hard into the floor so your shoulder blades kick out and your chest sinks (this is what gymnasts refer to as the hollow position). Tuck in your pelvis and flex your abs. Tense your whole body. Have your training partner lift your feet and then release one of them without warning. Your tightness should prevent your leg from falling. The partner must exercise caution and hold his hand a few inches below your ankle to prevent the leg from falling to the ground and breaking your toe should your tension be inadequate.

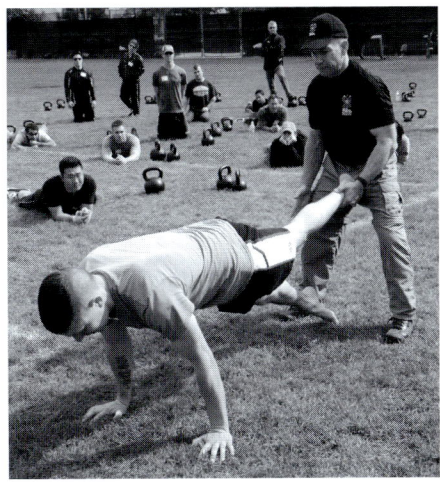

Elite gymnast and California bench press record-holder Mark Reifkind, Master RKC, is putting a student through the paces in the drop plank. The student has let his leg drop and is about face the consequences.

The next drill, also from Rif's toolbox, is the reverse drop plank. It should be obvious from the photo what you are supposed to do. (Just to be sure, you are lying on your back, again with your body tensed and a partner holding your feet off the ground. Try to keep your leg from dropping when it is suddenly released by keeping your body tight.)

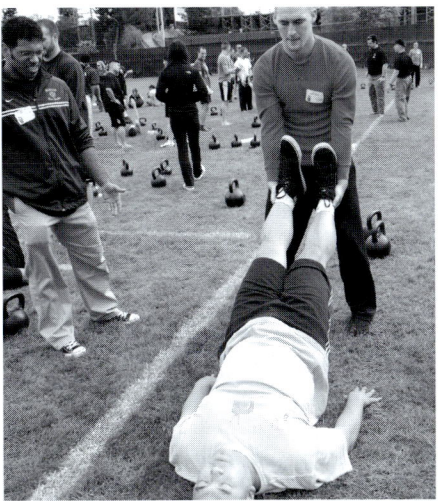

**The reverse drop plank.**

Zipping up is a pre-tension technique that will help you with your planks and with almost any lift. Pull up your kneecaps by tensing your quads. Now focus on pulling your quads up even higher into your groin, like window shutters.

Next do the same with the rest of your thigh muscles: the inner, the outer, and the hamstrings. It is as if you have grabbed your leg with both hands just above the knee, squeezed, and slowly pulled up all the thigh muscles into the groin. Imagine that you are sucking your hip joint into the hip socket as well.

The zipped-up feeling is very powerful. Your thigh muscles will feel very short, hard, and retracted into the pelvis.

Flex your glutes as if you are pinching a coin.

Work your way up your body—the waist is next. Shorten the muscles surrounding your waist—the abs, the obliques, the muscles around your ribs. Zip up all your torso muscles from your ribs down to your pelvis. Breathe shallowly as your respiratory muscles get constricted; do not hold your breath!

Flex the pecs and the lats so they pull your shoulders down, away from your ears. B. K. S. Iyengar, a yoga master, says that "the traps belong to the back, not the neck." Shorten your armpit muscles even further so they pull your shoulders into your body.

Pull your rigid arms into the shoulder sockets; retract them like telescopic antennae.

If you can figure out how, "screw" your shoulders into their sockets from inside out, right arm clockwise, left one counterclockwise.

Make the biceps and the triceps retreat into the deltoids. It is the same rolling up of the shades that you did with your thigh muscles.

Gather up your forearm muscles by your elbows and pull up your forearm bones into the elbows.

> ZIP!
> YOU HAVE ACHIEVED A VERY COMPACT AND POWERFUL ALIGNMENT.

Zip! You have achieved a very compact and powerful alignment.

These pre-tension techniques will make your body feel as hard and strong as steel. All the top guys are already doing this, whether they realize it or not. I hope this article will help you to reverse engineer their body language and strength.

Power to you! **M**

---

## The Best Workout Ever!

### Steve Jeck

Author of *The Stone Lifter* and
co-author of *Of Stones and Strength*

*"Nothing will work unless you do."*
—Maya Angelou

This I know . . .

You can be handed the best workout in the world and attack it with the intensity of limp lettuce and nothing will happen.

On the other hand, you can be handed the worst workout in the world and attack it with the intensity (as Doug Hepburn once described) of one charging into a machine gun turret and you will make great gains.

In other words, the workout itself is not the most crucial component in

> I'M GOING TO TAKE A SLIGHT DEPARTURE IN THIS *MILO* . . . GET DOWNRIGHT PRACTICAL BY DESCRIBING THE BEST WORKOUT I'VE EVER USED.

determining your training success; rather, it is your attitude and application of that workout that matters most.

Of course, it must be noted that the ultimate combination in guaranteeing training success would be to combine a great workout with a great approach—and then watch out, brother, it's ON . . . like Donkey Kong!

I'm going to take a slight departure in this *MILO* from focusing primarily on the mental arsenal side of the equation and get downright practical by describing the best workout I've ever used.

This workout (or some variation of it) is the program that I used during my competitive years in the Highland Games (1987–1997). It was also my workout of choice any time I set about on a stone lifting quest. Finally, these exercises, along with the suggested rep and set schemes, helped me maintain a pretty decent level of functional strength as I routinely hauled four boulders around the country in my 1992 Ford F150, ultimately giving over 100 stone lifting exhibitions between the years 1997–2007. Trust me, this program will work—IF YOU DO!

The workout, in a nutshell, consists of lifting three days a week—I have found a Mon–Thurs–Sat combo to be most effective. You will be squatting on Mondays and Thursdays, pairing a few "push" and "pull" movements respectively on those days; and Saturday will be devoted entirely to either "push" OR "pull" movements. I am using the quotation marks because I am aware of the fact that all muscles pull, not push; however, if you've been lifting for more than a week or two, you're well-versed in the weight room vernacular of push movements and pull movements so I am using these terms for reference sake (exercise science and physiology folks out there, cut me a little slack . . . thanks).

It is important to note that you will rotate your push and pull days each week, so that one week you will be pushing on Monday and Saturday, and pulling only on Thursday. The following week you will do your pulling movements on Monday and Saturday and pushing only on Thursday. The one constant is you will always squat on Monday and Thursday.

Having given you that overview, let's dig in and see what it should all look like.

**Week 1**

| Monday | Thursday | Saturday |
|---|---|---|
| Squats | Squats | Bench press |
| Incline bench | Power clean from hang | Incline DB press |
| Standing press | Cable rows | (Lat pulldown) |
| Dips | DB curls | Triceps pushdowns |

**Week 2**

| | | |
|---|---|---|
| Squats | Squats | Deadlifts |
| Barbell rows | Incline bench | Barbell rows |
| Power snatch from hang | Push press | (DB bench) |
| Heavy DB shrugs | Triceps pushdowns | Cable rows |
| Standing EZ bar curls | | |

For week three you will repeat week one, and for week four you will repeat week two, continuing that pattern.

A couple of things to note: You no doubt noticed that on Saturdays I've included a pull movement on your push day and a push movement on your pull day: the lat pulldowns and DB bench in parentheses. Even though these are primarily push or pull days, I've always found that throwing in the occasional alternate movement is great for muscle balance purposes; and it gives the pushing (or pulling) muscles a little breather.

You may also be wondering about the inclusion of cable rows, along with the triceps pushdowns and EZ curls. First of all, I'm not talking about performing the cable rows like most bodybuilders do, keeping the upper body perpendicular to the floor and basically just protracting and retracting the shoulder blades. That technique may be best for chiseling the rhomboids, but it will not make you big and strong. On the other hand, if you can work up to using the stack (and then pinning on a few extra 25-lb. plates) and exerting force through a full range of motion, performing most of your reps from good "at attention" posture but not being afraid to bend at the waist and reach for your toes, as well as throwing in a few hyperextensions in the mix; then you will develop boatloads of functional strength and split all of your blazers at the seams!

"That's fine, Steve, but what about the bi's and tri's? Now I know you're turning poser on me," you might be wondering, an understandable response. I have never advised against hitting a few arm movements, just not starting your workout with arms or worse yet, having an arms day! Arms are like dessert—as long as you've cleaned your plates (pun intended), you've earned the right to indulge a little. Or as Pink Floyd once said, "If you don't eat your meat, you can't have any pudding; how can you have any pudding if you don't eat your meat?"

Lastly, what about sets and reps? I will tell you what worked best for me.

> ARMS ARE LIKE DESSERT—AS LONG AS YOU'VE CLEANED YOUR PLATES (PUN INTENDED), YOU'VE EARNED THE RIGHT TO INDULGE A LITTLE.

As for the squats, I preferred 3 x 5 and then dropping 50 lb. and hitting a set of 10 (thank you, Jack King). You will need a few warm-up sets to climb up to those sets of 5, as they need to be heavy work sets, and even the dropdown set of 10 should be no walk in the park.

My benching sets (flat, incline or DB) usually looked something like 10, 8, 5, 5.

Power clean and snatch reps should be in the 3–5 range, 4–5 sets of each.

Barbell rows, you're looking at 4–5 sets, 5–7 reps.

Standing press and push press should be 5 x 5.

Cable rows and lat pulldowns should be 4 x 10.

And arms, who cares? Just feed the pythons until they're full!

There you have it, the Best Workout I've ever used. And it is guaranteed to work . . . IF YOU DO! M

# The Other Modern-Day Epidemic:

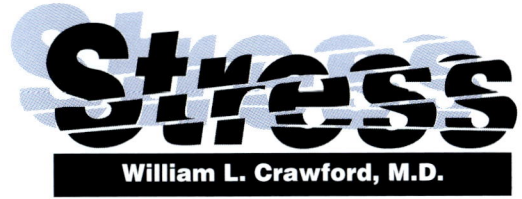

## Stress
### William L. Crawford, M.D.

Obesity is the most prevalent modern-day epidemic. What is second to obesity? Stress—the other modern-day epidemic that seems to be hidden in plain sight in our society these days. Stress can drive up blood pressure and promote cardiovascular disease, as well as cause a host of other physical and mental ailments. Most horrifying of all, stress can deter training progress, if not directly cause us to lose strength. Read on as we explore the physiologic effects of stress, the hidden signs of stress, and how to combat this silent killer.

Our bodies are built for stress. Our fight-or-flight response to stress is our "stand and fight" versus our "let's get the heck out of here" survival mechanism. This very basic system has allowed humans to adapt and survive for countless generations. The response is initiated in a deep brain structure known as the hypothalamus and is complemented by other brain stem structures.

The hypothalamus directs an outpouring of our sympathetic nervous system. This neurologically mediated response sets off a cascade of hormonal responses that include increased blood pressure, increased blood flow to the muscles, increased muscular strength, increased blood glucose concentrations, and heightened mental awareness. Sounds like getting psyched up for a big lift, doesn't it? This is not a bad thing—as a matter of fact, recent research has shown that some stress is good for our bodies and mental states. Stress offers the temporary benefits of keeping us physically and mentally sharp. However, because stress is like a hidden factor X that helps us maximize our capabilities to meet certain situations, we are also at risk if this system goes unchecked. Some stress is good but a continued level of stress over a period of time is detrimental.

> UNUSED BLOOD GLUCOSE IS TURNED TO FAT AND CAN ALSO CAUSE TRUNCAL OBESITY—IN OTHER WORDS A BIG GUT AND LOVE HANDLES

What does all this mean? Read on.

Stress increases cortisol levels and this in turn raises vascular tone. Simply put, hypertension can be a byproduct of prolonged stress. Heart disease, stroke, and kidney failure are among the prime problems that are caused by hypertension. Overeating and poor sleep caused by stress can promote obesity. Also, blood glucose levels can be increased with prolonged stress through release of glucose stores from the liver, a main area of glucose storage and production. A relative diabetic state can ensue. Unused blood glucose is turned to fat and can also cause truncal obesity—in other words a big gut and love handles.

Body fat stores in the trunk have been correlated to increased risks of cardiac events—or again simply put, a heart attack. Getting the point?

Insomnia and mental irritability also are byproducts of prolonged stress. Want to derail yourself at home and at work? Be a stressed-out maniac for a while and see what that does for your personal and professional life.

What are we to do? Quit our jobs, tell our bosses to take a hike, or tell our kids good luck in raising themselves? Of course not. But stress is with us. What if you find yourself miserable or even on medications to combat hypertension, anxiety, or depression because you are stressed?

As a MILO reader you have one of the best ways to fight stress at your disposal: exercise. But is that enough? Not completely, but it certainly is a giant step forward.

Let me go off course here for a minute and then get back to exercise as a way to fight stress. Studies have shown that meditation has actually been used to get people off blood pressure medications. You don't have to turn into a guru or move to a mountain top to contemplate the mysteries of life. As a simple way to relax, or more accurately meditate on relaxing, try this simple exercise. Sit in a quiet, comfortable place or even lie down. Close your eyes and focus on breathing in and out until you establish a steady, relaxed breathing pattern. Now, take a deep breath and hold it for about 10 seconds and subsequently let the breath out slowly. After the exhalation, forcibly exhale and hold that exhalation for about 10 seconds. Repeat the cycle 3 to 5 times.

Resume the slow, steady breaths and begin focusing on relaxing each individual muscle group. Start with the facial muscles, letting the muscles in your face go slack. Move down the body to the traps, pectorals, lats, and abdominal muscles, and on down to your feet. You want the sensation of deep relaxation, even heaviness.

In this state of relaxation, continue to focus on your breathing. Visualize the air moving in and out of your lungs; go to a place in your mind and think about your next training session, maximizing the benefit of your deep state of relaxation. See yourself going to the gym, selecting an exercise, warming up, and successfully completing your workout weight by weight and set by set. This technique will enhance your training sessions. In other words, you will be using the relaxed state to fuel your training; that training can, in turn, relieve your stress—a win-win situation if ever there was one.

Using this relaxation technique can help you sleep as well. Sleep can also combat stress and all the ills that come with it. Our friend and esteemed strength authority Bill Starr has written about a natural substance called dolomite or calcium-magnesium tablets to aid in sleep. Take a couple of these tablets before bed with a little milk and this combination of minerals will potentiate the nervous system to relax. I dream very vividly when I use this brain-relaxing mineral combo. Plus, calcium and magnesium are used by our bodies in many positive ways. Another win-win situation.

> I FIND THAT THROWING HIGHLAND GAMES IMPLEMENTS PUTS ME IN A MORE UPBEAT AND RELAXED STATE OF MIND.

Now back to exercise. Lifting heavy weights is a great stress reliever. I find that throwing Highland Games implements puts me in a more upbeat and relaxed state of mind. A good walk, tossing the ball with my kids, or throwing a ball to my dog helps as well, but exercise is the key ingredient.

I know this is preaching to the choir. As a MILO reader you are a different breed and likely train hard with little or no prompting. What does this mean to you in terms of exercise? Sure, a big set of squats is helpful, but a drop-back set is beneficial to get your heart rate up a bit more. I have written about the drop-back set with squats showing a positive cardiovascular training effect. This is a set of 10 to 20 reps with 50% to 70% of the weight you finished with your top working set. For example, if you performed a set of 5 with 300 lb. for your working weight with your squats, dropping back to 150 to 200 lb. for a set of 10 to 20 reps would provide a cardiovascular training benefit. How do you feel after those 20 reps? As Steve Jeck said on his *Cellar Dwellers* DVD after performing a set of 25 reps with 225 lb. on the bench press, "I feel at peace with my fellow man."

Not to sound like a broken record from my prior articles in MILO, cardiovascular training is also a great stress reliever. Walking, jogging, Battling Ropes, striking a tire with a sledgehammer, hitting a heavy bag, the list is endless. Get your heart rate up for 30 minutes, 3 times per week, and it is like money in the bank for providing stress-relieving workouts. Since getting more serious about cardiovascular work over the last year, I have lost some weight but my strength levels remain high. Quite frankly, as well being in better physical condition, I sleep better and feel less on edge.

Stress is a breeding ground for anxiety, and anxiety in turn is a close cousin to depression. That's right, stress can lead to depression. Think about it: if your motor is running at a higher baseline than normal, at some point your brain and body may not be able to continue to keep pace. You will run low on the chemicals that sustain a healthy state of mind. Depression is a serious medical condition but it can be avoided or promptly treated if recognized early enough. Symptoms of depression can be loss of enjoyment in your usual activities, loss of libido, and sleeping more or less than usual, to name a few. There are several websites that can give more details about more subtle features of depression and of course you should always call your physician to discuss signs of depression and its treatment. Why bring this up in a strength journal? It's hard to be strong physically when your state of mind is suffering. Depression is not a weakness and is a treatable condition.

> STRESS IS A BREEDING GROUND FOR ANXIETY, AND ANXIETY IN TURN IS A CLOSE COUSIN TO DEPRESSION.

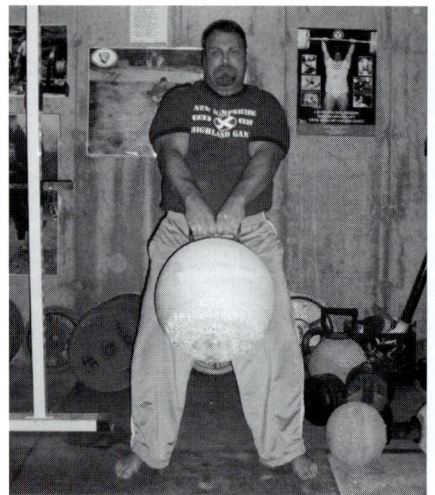
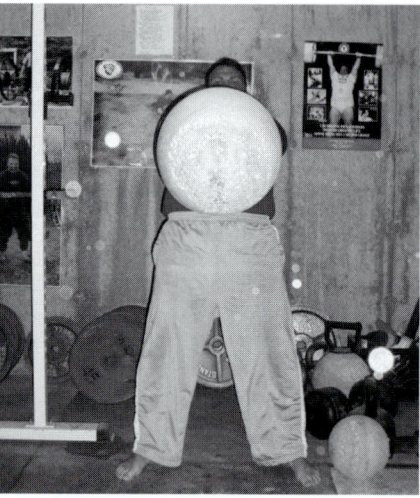

Talk about stress relief! Try swinging a 175-lb. stone kettleball 10 times.

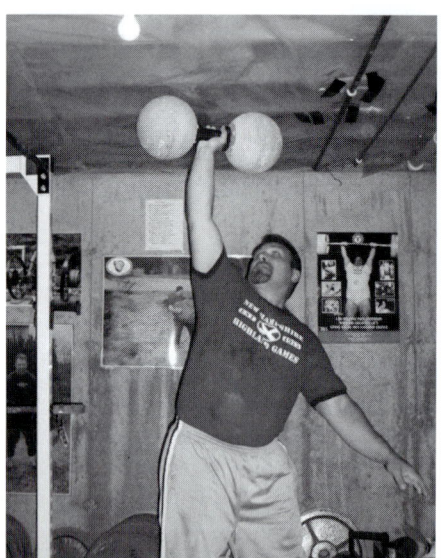

Lifting a 3-in.-handled dumbbell made with a 60-lb. stone ball on each end, total weight 125 lb., can help put things in perspective.
Holly Crawford photos.

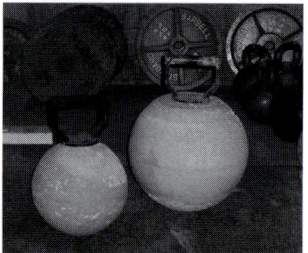

A 100-lb. kettleball and the 175-lb. kettleball in repose. Steve Slater molds and handles.

Can stress kill you? Of course it can. There are countless cases of people receiving bad news and having a fatal heart attack or stroke. More insidious are the cases of people who silently languish in a state of stress and anxiety, which slowly leads to serious, and eventually fatal, conditions.

Let's move on from the doom and gloom to focus on your training. A state of mind that is clouded can be helped with a tough training session.

But if you are having a hard time sleeping or if you generally lack energy because your life is overwhelming you, your brain and neurologic system becomes drained, which takes away your edge. Poor training or poor focus can lead to frustration and, worse yet, an injury. I have looked at my training logs and see periods of plateaus in training or even steps backward in strength gains that correlate well with times of personal stress.

Most of us are self-motivated, focused, over-the-top sorts of guys—but don't think that stress can't catch up with you. Get a good night's sleep, eat properly, try meditating, and train, train, train. Most importantly, keep the balance in your life. If work is taking loads of time and energy, continue your training but consider that maybe you need to switch gears and do something a little differently. I train at home for many reasons, but the prime consideration is that my schedule is very erratic. Training at 5 a.m., 10 p.m., or at any available time is an option for me.

Try some bodyweight exercises once in a while, or only use dumbbells in a training session. Modifying sets, reps, and exercises can set you up to have a heavier workout down the road if you are wise about your choices. Live to fight another day—the point is to keep the training ball rolling. Truthfully, don't you feel better after any workout? A kettlebell or a grip training workout is a favorite of mine if I am pressed for time. If I have been working overnights or evenings, I reduce the weight handled in a routine by 10% and stick with less technically difficult exercises, such as high pulls instead of snatches. This is being practical, as neuromuscular coordination is hampered if I am off my usual rest schedule.

My previous article about daily hormone levels and training times ["Training by Your Body Clock," MILO June 2010, Vol. 18, No. 1] explains how to modify your training to meet the demands of life. That doesn't mean you can just give up and not train hard. Much to the contrary, you are trying to tailor the realities of your life to continue to make progress.

Take the burden of a hard day and turn it into fuel for a great workout. Seriously, I have sometimes dedicated my top set to an event of the day or to someone who wasn't as cordial in their dealings with me as I would have liked. Okay, flat tire, here is a set of 20-rep squats just for you! I literally visualize the freezing cold highway, fumbling with a set of directions in 8 languages to figure out the Gordian knot of the tire jack in my mini-van . . . ohhhhh . . . blast off!

> LIVE TO FIGHT ANOTHER DAY— THE POINT IS TO KEEP THE TRAINING BALL ROLLING.

Again, as Professor Jeck said after his high-rep set, "I feel at peace with my fellow man." Work actively to keep your stress levels manageable and you will reap the benefits in your health, your personal life, and your training. And isn't that what this is all about anyway?

# Foundations:
## Controlled Striking for Physical and Mental Toughness

### Jon Bruney

**M**ILO readers understand that making gains in strength requires a certain amount of discomfort. We want to train the body by overloading it with exercise in hopes that it will adapt and be stronger. Repeated stress causes muscle, ligament, and bone adaptation. One of the unique ways this can be accomplished is through the discipline of iron body or controlled striking. Conditioning the body to withstand the impact of being struck repeatedly by different implements in a controlled manner will cause the muscles to become harder, stronger, and more resilient. Teaching the body to absorb impact will also benefit athletes who compete in combat sports, such as football, hockey, and MMA.

This article is a brief overview of how you can apply striking to your workouts—it will only scratch the surface of this powerful discipline. I am not an iron body expert, but I have been using different striking exercises in my training for a long time. I will not get into the different *qi qong* exercises that accompany the martial art of iron body. I will be focusing on the striking exercises that can be used to increase strength and mental toughness.

> . . . MAKING GAINS IN STRENGTH REQUIRES A CERTAIN AMOUNT OF DISCOMFORT.

To practice iron body effectively, you will need some kind of implement to strike your body with. The most common are the iron hammer and the beating bag. I use both of these implements regularly. The iron hammer is a long piece of wood with several slats carved into it, which help to absorb some of the impact of the strike. The hammer makes a slapping sound as it hits your body. The beating bag is made of canvas and is usually filled with mung beans for beginners. Advanced athletes have beating bags filled with smooth stones.

Once you have obtained your implements, you are ready to begin. I recommend that you practice iron body techniques at the end of your strength training workouts. Starting at the forearms, take the hammer or the bag in one hand and begin to strike the other arm. The strike should be hard enough to cause a slight sting in the beginning. Each strike should be under control. Be careful not to injure yourself by striking too hard—the idea is to cause repeated stress on the body, not injury. Repeatedly strike the forearms on all sides for at least 20 seconds. As you get stronger, you can increase the time. Continue to strike the rest of the body, moving to the upper arms, shoulders, chest, abdominals, and legs. You should feel invigorated after your iron body practice.

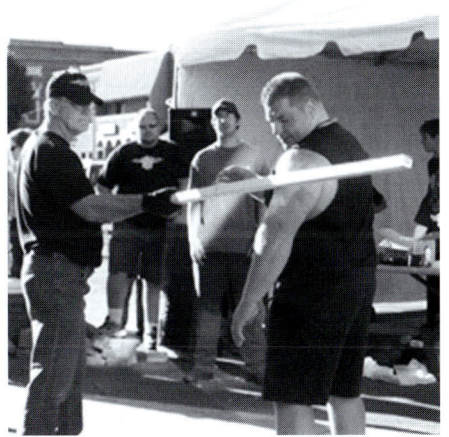

*Jon, ready to have a board broken across his shoulder.*

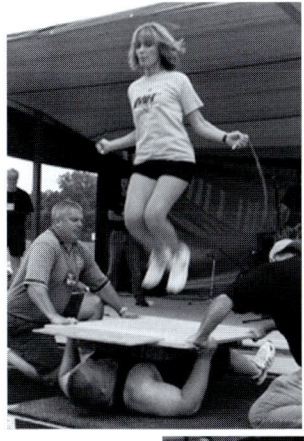

**Supporting a bed of nails and jumper.**

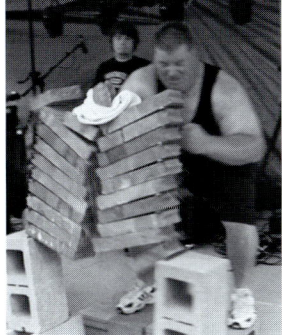

**Breaking a stack of concrete bricks.**
Erica Renee photos.

Most iron body practitioners recommend applying *dit da jow* after training. I occasionally will do this. The *dit da jow* is a liniment that will help to toughen the skin and help heal bruises. In my opinion, Tiger Balm and Icy Hot work well, too.

As you continue the practice of iron body, you will notice some changes in your body. The muscles will feel denser. I have observed that my tendons are stronger. You will also be tougher mentally—repeated striking definitely builds mental toughness—and you will have higher pain tolerance.

I can attest to the fact that basic iron body training works. I have boards broken over my arms in my strongman shows (see this YouTube video for an example: http://www.youtube.com/watch?v=tZMJEWmBGSs). I am able to break boards and bricks with my hands. I also have learned to absorb impact. One of the feats in my shows involves my lying under a bed of nails while my wife jumps rope on top of me. Iron body work has been a major key to performing these feats.

Give this basic training a try; you'll be glad you did. Again, this is not an article on the traditional martial art of iron body. There are many books and DVDs that teach traditional iron body. My goal is to show how strength athletes can use the controlled striking exercise from the iron body discipline to become stronger. This article presents the basics only. Use this article wisely—you must be responsible for your iron body work and be sure to not injure yourself. Best of luck with your training. **M**

# It's Never Too Late

## Jim Schmitz
U.S. Olympic Team Weightlifting Coach 1980, 1988, & 1992

I've had some incredible experiences in my years in the strength and health business, coaching and watching the best weightlifters in the United States and the world. What I would like to share in this article are some very impressive weightlifting results by older men and women. I'm not going to talk about guys like Mike Huszka, Walt Imahara, and Fred Lowe who were really strong as young men as well as when they were older. Rather, I'm going to talk about men and women who took up weightlifting later in life, after their prime athletic years. I define these from 15 to 30 years old, which is when most athletes have their greatest success.

One of the most famous older strongmen was Karl Norberg. Karl is a whole article in his own right, and I have talked about Karl in previous *MILO* articles, but the short summary is that he took up weightlifting at age 68 when he retired from being a San Francisco longshoreman and Alaska fisherman. At 73 years old he bench pressed 460 lb. (208 kg); at 80 he could still do 400 lb. (181 kg); and at 85 he could still do 300 lb. (136 kg). Karl weighed around 255 lb. (116 kg) during those years.

Next is Dan Takeuchi. I wrote a *MILO* article about him a year or so ago ["My Grandfather Can Outlift Yours—and You, Too! The Dan Takeuchi Story," September 2008, Vol. 16, No. 2]. His story is similar to Karl's. Dan took up Olympic-style weightlifting when he retired from being a truck driver and farmer at age 54. He went on to win the Masters' World Championships and set many masters' world records. He cleaned and jerked 225 lb. (102.5 kg) at 70 years old and did 194 lb. (88 kg) at age 80 at a bodyweight of 165 to 170 lb. (75 to 77 kg).

Bob Strange is another who took up Olympic-style weightlifting when he retired at age 58, but he didn't have a physically demanding job. Bob actually took up weight training at age 45 and got into powerlifting at age 49. It turned out that Bob had a lot of natural strength he just hadn't used yet. He grew up on a farm in Oregon and never touched a weight until he was a freshman in college, when he military pressed his bodyweight (around 180 lb. /81.5 kg) in order to get an 'A' in a physical education class. At 58 he began Olympic lifting because he met and trained with Don Ramos, a world champion masters' lifter. Bob's best powerlifts were: squat 551 lb. (250 kg) at age 58 and 198 lb. (90 kg) bodyweight; bench press 375 lb. (170 kg) at age 59 and 207 lb. (94 kg) bodyweight; and deadlift 601 lb. (272.5 kg) at age 60 and 207 lb. (94 kg) bodyweight. His best Olympic lifts were: snatch 92.5 kg (204 lb.) at age 63 and 93.2 kg (205 lb.) bodyweight; and clean and jerk 120 kg (264 lb.) at age 64 and 91.6 kg (202 lb.) bodyweight. Now at 73 years old and

91.5 kg (201.5 lb.), he still does a 75-kg (165-lb.) snatch and 95-kg (209-lb.) clean and jerk—very impressive lifting in both strength sports. Another thing about Bob is that he looks at least 20 years younger than he is and he is fast, strong, and very athletic.

Arnie Lazarus joined my gym to lose weight and get in shape when he was 61 years old. He was watching the weightlifters work out and asked me if he could do it. I told him to come back and see me when he could back squat 135 lb. (61 kg) for 3 sets of 10 reps. That was a method I used to weed out the serious and not-so-serious. In two months he came back, said he could do it, and showed me an easy 10 reps with 132 lb. (60 kg)—so I started him on my raw beginner Olympic-style weightlifting program, which consists of the power clean from the thighs, clean deadlift and shrug, push press, and back squat. He could barely deadlift 132 lb. (60 kg) for 5 reps, but I started him off with very light weights and he plugged away. After a couple of months I had him doing hang power snatches, power cleans from the floor, push jerks, clean deadlift and shrugs, and back squats and front squats. After another few months I had him doing split snatches and split clean and jerks, as he didn't have the flexibility for squat snatches and squat cleans.

After a year or so he wanted to see what he could do in competition, so he entered the 2003 Golden West Open and did a 45-kg (99-lb.) snatch and a 60-kg (132-lb.) clean and jerk at 84 kg (185 lb.) bodyweight. Unfortunately in this first contest he developed a hernia, but he had it repaired and returned to training after three months.

> ANOTHER THING ABOUT BOB IS THAT HE LOOKS AT LEAST 20 YEARS YOUNGER THAN HE IS AND HE IS FAST, STRONG, AND VERY ATHLETIC.

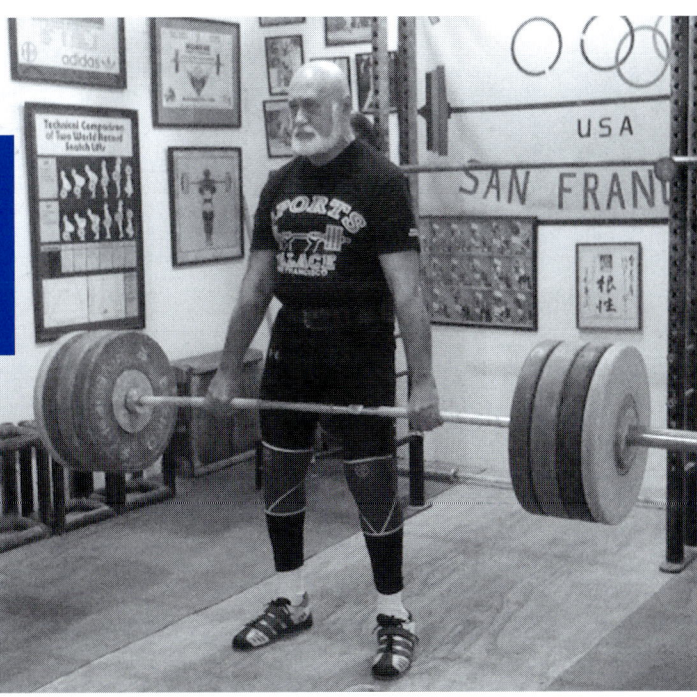

Arnie Lazarus lifting 182.4 kg (402 lb.) at age 67 and a bodyweight of 85 kg (187 lb.).
Jim Schmitz photo.

Arnie continued to train and improve, but his lack of flexibility was his main problem, although it did improve considerably. His best snatch was 50 kg (110 lb.) and his best clean and jerk was 68 kg (150 lb.) at a bodyweight of 85 kg (187 lb.) at age 66. Arnie did find out, however, that he could deadlift and squat some pretty impressive weights. He deadlifted 182.5 kg (402 lb.) and back squatted 125 kg (275 lb.), also at 85 kg bodyweight at age 67. Those weights may not sound impressive to *MILO* readers, but considering where he started (and if you saw him) you would lose a lot of money if you bet against him deadlifting. Butch Curry, 1980 Olympian, called Arnie a deadlift *savant* because Arnie in no way shape or form looks as if he could deadlift over 400 lb. (182.5 kg). He looks more like a retired college professor than a weightlifter.

> THERE ARE SEVERAL WOMEN WHOM I HAVE HELPED START LIFTING LATER IN THEIR ATHLETIC LIVES, AND THEY HAVE DONE SOME PRETTY IMPRESSIVE LIFTING.

There are several women whom I have helped start lifting later in their athletic lives, and they have done some pretty impressive lifting. Anne Lehman began Olympic lifting at age 34. Her best lifts were: snatch 58 kg (128 lb.), clean and jerk 77.5 kg (171 lb.), squat 115 kg (253 lb.), and deadlift 115 kg (253 lb.) at 58 kg (128 lb.) bodyweight and 45 years old. She has qualified and competed in several American Opens and U.S. National Championships where she is quite often over twice the age of the lifters she is out-performing. Anne cleans up in masters' competition where she has set records in different age groups and bodyweight classes and has won the outstanding lifter award for women of all ages and bodyweights at the National Masters' and World Masters' competitions. Now at age 50 she has qualified for the U.S. Nationals again. She has dropped down to the 48-kg (106-lb.) class as her lifts are coming down with age, but she is still competitive in the lighter weight class.

Jennifer Kanenaga took up weight training to get stronger in order to be an emergency medical technician. She was 34 years old, 4' 11", and 50 kg (110 lb.) when she started. After a few months of weight training and seeing women doing Olympic lifting, she asked if she could try it. She did and got quite good, with best lifts of snatch 57 kg (125.5 lb.), clean and jerk 64 kg (141 lb.), and back squat 88 kg (194 lb.) at age 42 and 48 kg (106 lb.) bodyweight. She has won several National Masters' Championships and set many masters' records, and she placed second at the 2009 U.S. National Championships in the 48-kg class at 42 years of age.

JoAnn Arnold started Olympic lifting at 33 years old because soon after she joined my gym to get back into shape, she saw other women doing weightlifting and wanted to try it. After a couple of years we talked her into competing and she now has best lifts of 61 kg (134 lb.) in the snatch, 81 kg (178.5 lb.) in the clean and jerk, and 115 kg (253 lb.) in the back squat at 53 kg (117 lb.) at 39 years old. JoAnn has placed fourth at the American Open and U.S. Nationals, just missing third place by bodyweight, or a kilo or two. To show how dedicated she is to her lifting, she would bring her six-month-old baby to the gym and nurse him in between sets.

Julia Jung-Ames took up Olympic-style weightlifting at age 47 on the recommendation of her inline skating coach, Sandy Snakenberg. She just did the Olympic lifts, plus pulls and squats, to improve her strength and power for skating and bicycling. She trained pretty hard and lifted pretty good weights. A few days after her fiftieth birthday she cleaned and jerked 45.5 kg (100 lb.) at a bodyweight of 59 kg (130 lb.). I and the women on my team finally talked her into competing and she did very well and now competes regularly. Her best lifts are snatch 36 kg (79 lb.), clean and jerk 50 kg (110 lb.), back squat 65 kg (143 lb.), and deadlift 81 kg (178 lb.) at 59 kg (130 lb.) bodyweight and 54 years old. Julia power snatches and power cleans due to tender knees—she has a lot of explosive power.

Kathy Mitchell began Olympic lifting at age 51 because her son is a CrossFit coach and he thought it would be good for her. The squat snatch and squat clean come quite naturally to Kathy. It's quite rare for a 50-year-old to be able to do full rock-bottom squat snatches and cleans, but Kathy has no problem and her knees don't suffer at all. She has very good technique in the snatch and the clean, but her jerk is a problem because her legs need to be stronger. Kathy's best lifts are snatch 35 kg (77 lb.), clean and jerk 44 kg (97 lb.), back squat 60 kg (132 lb.), and deadlift 75 kg (165 lb.) at 60 kg (132 lb.) bodyweight and 54 years old.

There may be many women out there who took up weightlifting later in their athletic lives and who lift more weight than the women I have mentioned above, but these are the women I know and have trained, so I have firsthand knowledge of their training and competing. Think of your mother or even grandmother lifting those weights!

I do personal training at the Claremont Country Club in Oakland, just across the bay from San Francisco. This country club is primarily for socializing, golf, and tennis, but they do have a very nice weight room with a good platform and barbell set. Hank Carlson started working out with me when he was 67; he had only been doing weight training for a couple of years after about 40-plus years of no weight training, although he did do a lot of running and played golf. Hank wanted to learn how to do the snatch and clean and jerk so we started working together about two years ago. Now at age 69, he can power snatch 50 kg (110 lb.), clean and jerk 66 kg (145 lb.), and deadlift 113 kg (250 lb.) x 2 at a bodyweight of 81.6 kg (180 lb.). His snatch and clean are done in the power style as he doesn't have the flexibility to do a full squat. Hank really likes the movements of the snatch and clean and jerk, and he understands that they really work the entire body completely.

I began training Ed Bartlett, another Claremont Country Club member, when he was 77 years old. Ed had played football at the University of California at Berkeley (1949, 1950, and 1951) where he played defensive end and was named to the All-Pac 8 (now Pac 10), received an honorable mention as an All-American, and played in the College All-Star Game and two Rose Bowls in 1950 and 1951. He didn't lift weights then, as very few did, and he didn't do anything really physical for about 53 years until he started weight training with me. He worked out as hard as he felt comfortable and got up to some respectable weights, outlifting men twenty years his junior. For example, he could do lat pulldowns with 180 lb. (81 kg) and dumbbell curl and press 10 lb. (4.5 kg). He also lost 40 lb. since we have been working together. Ed just does weight training, stretching, and walking, but he does a very substantial workout. Although he isn't impressed with his workouts, I am because the older you get, the harder it gets. Of course at 82 years of age there is a little drop-off, but he is still doing a very respectable workout.

Now Ed and Hank are no Bob Strange, Dan Takeuchi, or Karl Norberg, but I mention them to show that no matter what your age or physical condition, it is never too late to take up serious weightlifting or weight training.

One more person of note is Pax Beale. Pax just turned 80 and looks at least 20 years younger. Pax was an athlete pretty much all his life, playing football and throwing the shot and discus in high school and college; he also boxed professionally for a few years, and then was a competitive distance runner for many years. However, he never really worked out with the weights. At 52 years old he took up bodybuilding and really got into it, winning many masters' titles, and now at 80, he looks, moves, and talks like someone half his age.

> MOST PEOPLE THEIR AGES WOULD SAY, "I'M TOO OLD FOR WEIGHTLIFTING, I'LL DO SOMETHING LESS STRENUOUS LIKE SWIMMING, CARDIO MACHINES, PILATES, OR YOGA."

It's very interesting that the twelve people mentioned took up weight training and weightlifting later in life and wanted be strong as well as healthy and fit. Most people their ages would say, "I'm too old for weightlifting, I'll do something less strenuous like swimming, cardio machines, Pilates, or yoga." I don't want to take anything away from any other physical training methods; they all are excellent. It's just that I've been lifting heavy weights for fifty years—and coaching people to lift heavy weights for forty years—and I believe it is the best way to train. Being strong and powerful, as well as healthy and fit, is the best—no matter how old you are. I am very glad that more and more people are "getting it" and realizing that it feels good to be strong and lift heavy weights.

## Getting started

How do you go about heavy weightlifting later in your life? Remember, heavy is relative, it is whatever is heavy for you. First you have to have the desire and will. Then it is best to have a qualified and experienced coach or trainer. Beware of trainers who want to push too hard, and make sure you go at your own pace. Begin with very light weights and work on improving your form and increasing your workout capacity. As important as your form or technique is, you have to go with the best you can do.

> WITH AGE WE LOSE OUR FLEXIBILITY, SPEED, AND COORDINATION— THEY CAN BE IMPROVED, BUT IT TAKES TIME, PATIENCE, AND PERSISTENCE.

With age we lose our flexibility, speed, and coordination—they can be improved, but it takes time, patience, and persistence. You have to spend a lot of time stretching and doing technique work with a broomstick and empty barbell to improve your skills. The best way to lift weights is by using proper technique and form, but as we age, we just can't do things as well as we used to; that is a fact of life. Despite this, you still must always be working on and concentrating on your lifting technique because you want it to be as good as it can be. Instead of doing full squat snatches and cleans, maybe it's best to do power snatches or power cleans; or, (and I'm a big supporter of this) perform the split-style snatch and split-style clean. Maybe you can do only partial lifts like pulls, shrugs, lifting off blocks, quarter- or half-squats, and overhead lifts that don't lock out. Do whatever works best for you.

You have to let your progress happen or evolve, you can't push it. I like to call my training programs for older lifters the "enough" program; that is, you always train just "enough," whatever that is for you. Do just enough exercises, reps, sets, and weight—you want to walk out of the gym feeling good, not beat up or dead tired.

The most important factor for success for older lifters is consistency. You absolutely must train consistently—at least two times per week, maybe three, but no more than three weight workouts. You can do other things, such as cardio, on other days if you like and have the time and energy. After 50 years of age, though, most of us can only handle two to three weight workouts per week. The lifts, reps, sets, and weight will always vary, but you should try to do a pull, squat, and push in each workout. Also, the intensity and volume need to be fairly low and will vary from workout to workout. Older lifters can't train by percentages because they are too hard to predict as we are declining in strength whether we like it or not, and we are just trying to slow the process. If you try to train by percentages, you will definitely overtrain or injure yourself.

> THE MOTTO OF THE OLDER LIFTER SHOULD BE IF IT FEELS GOOD, DO IT; IF IT DOESN'T, DON'T!

Instead of using percentages, use the light, medium and heavy concept. For example one workout can be medium, the next workout light, the next workout heavy, and the next workout light; then repeat. Again what are light, medium, and heavy is totally up to you. Don't go heavy too often, maybe once a week or once every two weeks.

The motto of the older lifter should be if it feels good, do it; if it doesn't, don't! You are going to have workouts where nothing feels good—don't worry about it, save yourself for another day. Also, you will have workouts where everything feels great and you can lift all your weights and maybe even a little more with no problem. Enjoy these workouts—they happen only once in a while. Sometimes you might have several in a row, but be aware that great workouts don't happen every time, just from time to time.

Layoffs due to family, job, health, and life in general are a fact of life for the older lifter, so learn how to use them to your best advantage. If you know you have to take a layoff for whatever reason, train a little harder than normal, slightly overtraining so your body will need the rest. If you are really feeling beat up, tired and unmotivated, a layoff of a week or two might be just what you need. Unless you are ill, layoffs should be active rest periods of at least walking and stretching. When you come back from a layoff you will probably feel really good and want to train hard and heavy. Don't do it! Come back nice and easy, taking about two or three weeks to get back up to normal, whatever that is for you.

To give you an idea of how to balance your workouts, here are two sample Olympic lifting programs for the over-50 crowd. You may even want to do some bodybuilding exercises as well, which I think is good. Do them at the end of the workout or on alternate days and light for two to three sets of 10 reps. Forget about Chinese or Bulgarian programs or the famous Russian squat routine—their lifters began training around 10 to 12 years old and were selected, recruited, and rewarded.

Each workout must begin with a thorough and complete stretch, warm-up, and abdominal routine of 15 to 30 minutes. The actual lifting should last about 60 to 90 minutes at a reasonable pace, with 1- to 3-minute breaks between sets and exercises. Each workout should end with more stretching and abdominal work. Cardio and other physical activities should be done on alternate days or after the weight workout. I want to stress that some form of cardio (20 to 30 minutes) is an absolute must for the older strength athlete, as is stretching—do not neglect these two areas!

As important as your workouts are, so is your recovery. You have to get enough sleep and proper nutrition; in other words, adhere to very healthy living habits. Massage and sauna are

---

### Two Olympic lifting programs for +50-year-olds

**S** = snatch of any style—power, squat or split
**SHP** = snatch high pull or snatch pull of your choice
**BS** = back squat
**C&J** = clean & jerk of any style—power, squat or split
**CHP** = clean high pull or clean pull of your choice
**FS** = front squat
**CDL&S** = clean deadlift & shrug

**Two workouts per week:**

(A) Monday or Tuesday

Stretch – warm-up – abs
S       3x3 – 2 – 2 – 1 – 1
SHP     2 – 2 – 2
C&J     3x3 – 2 – 3x1
BS      5 – 4 – 3 – 2 – 1
Stretch, abs

(B) Friday or Saturday

Stretch – warm-up – abs
C&J     3x3 – 2 – 1 – 1 – 1
CDL&S   2 – 2 – 2
S       3x3 – 2 – 3x2
FS      5 – 4 – 3 – 2 – 1
Stretch, abs

**Three workouts per week:**

(A) Monday or Tuesday

Stretch – warm-up – abs
S       3x3 – 2 – 3x2
SHP     2 – 2 – 2
BS      5 – 4 – 3 – 2 – 1
Stretch, abs

(B) Wednesday or Thursday

Stretch – warm-up – abs
C&J     3x3 – 2 – 3x1
CHP     2 – 2 – 2
FS      5 – 4 – 3 – 2 – 1
Stretch, abs

(C) Friday or Saturday

Stretch – warm-up – abs
S       3x3 – 2 – 2 – 1 – 1
C&J     3x3 – 2 – 1 – 1 – 1
CDL&S   2 – 2 – 2
Stretch, abs

excellent for recovery. For sore muscles and joints, aspirin, ibuprofen, ice, and analgesic creams or liniments are the best. Fish oil, Omega-3 fatty acids, and glucosamine and/or chondroitin sulfate are also very good for the joints, tendons, and ligaments. Don't take powerful drugs to mask injuries or pain. Older athletes must listen to their pains and surrender to them. Pain is your yellow blinking light, meaning proceed with caution. If you were to mask a slight injury, you could make it a very serious injury. As we get older we have more aches and pains than when we were younger—that's just a fact of life. We have to listen to our bodies and always proceed accordingly. This doesn't mean you lie down and do nothing: life really is about using it or losing it, whether it's physical or mental capabilities. When working out, you have to train as hard as you feel good doing, but you must know when to say, "Enough!" Also, if you are on any medications, you really must check with your doctor about your exercise program. Just because you are feeling good doesn't mean you should go off your medications without consulting your doctor.

I have written three MILO articles for the older strength athlete. You might want to go back and read them for more information on the subject. The caveat is that those articles were written for strength athletes who have continued to lift and train all their lives:

- "Power Training for the +35-year-old Strength Athlete," December 1999, Vol. 7, No. 3
- "Five, Four, Three, Two, One—Done!" March 2000, Vol. 7, No 4
- "Once Strong, Twice Weak," December 2004, Vol. 12, No 3

There is a good book by Brooks D. Kubik called *Gray Hair and Black Iron*, which is about successful strength training for older lifters. I think it is a must-read for any lifter 50 years and over.

Sooner or later what goes up must come down. All of the people I have mentioned in this article will experience losing the ability to lift the weights they have built themselves up to lift, if they have not already. Don't quit when you start losing it; instead, continue to train as hard as you comfortably can. We want to slow down the aging process and stretch out the downward slope. Lifting whatever and however you can is good for you. You will get discouraged from time to time, but don't quit.

Remember, it's not how much you lift, but that fact that you *can* lift! Snatching and cleaning and jerking is fun and makes you feel good and look good, and you will be strong, fit and healthy. The ultimate goal is to maintain your strength, stamina, and suppleness for as long as possible, and then some! It's never too late to start.

> DON'T TAKE POWERFUL DRUGS TO MASK INJURIES OR PAIN. OLDER ATHLETES MUST LISTEN TO THEIR PAINS AND SURRENDER TO THEM.

## A Neglected King of Middleweight:

# Miro Gamba

### Gherardo Bonini

In the second half of the 1890s, European weightlifting had become quite widespread, especially in middle Europe. In the previous years, most of the lifters were corpulent and overweight athletes, naturally gifted for strength sports. But increasingly the number of weightlifters, especially middleweight and lightweight lifters, grew and logically also their performances. In the world championships in Amsterdam in April 1896, two lifters under 80 kg—the Italian Monticelli Obizzi and the Dutchman Philipp De Haas—challenged the heavier lifters and they performed very well.

In 1899, the English Amateur Gymnastic Association (AGA) organised for the first time a national championships with three bodyweight classes: lightweight, middleweight, and heavyweight. In the successive years, Austria (1901), France (1903), Germany (1905), and Italy (1907) also introduced these classes. Although there were some minor differences, the leading weightlifting countries settled on 70 kg as the limit for the lightweight class and 80 kg as that for the middleweight. Several good athletes belonging to these two classes competed and did not receive adequate honours. In Italy, Miro Gamba was one of them.

Gamba was born in Bellagio, near Como, Lombardy, on 14 August 1879. He completed his higher studies first in Pavia, and then in Turin, where in 1902 he obtained a diploma as an engineer at the prestigious Polytechnic University. It should be noted that Gamba became one of the most acclaimed professors of the university and a famous engineer, but his fame as a lifter was neglected.

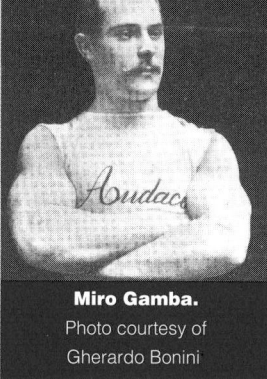

**Miro Gamba.**
Photo courtesy of Gherardo Bonini

Gamba made his debut in 1901, winning the Piedmont championships. On that occasion, he jerked with two hands 120 kg, improving to 125 in 1902 and 130 in 1903, always in the continental style, at a bodyweight of around 72 to 75 kg. In 1903, he pressed in the very clean style 107 kg—a sensational performance for a middleweight, as heavyweight athletes like Maspoli and Bonnes boasted 110 and 111, respectively. In total, Gamba won seven Piedmont championships and on these occasions he accomplished very good performances, but because the Italian gymnastics federation was the supervising body, his records were not recognized by the proper Italian

> IN 1903, HE PRESSED IN THE VERY CLEAN STYLE 107 KG—A SENSATIONAL PERFORMANCE FOR A MIDDLEWEIGHT, AS HEAVYWEIGHT ATHLETES LIKE MASPOLI AND BONNES BOASTED 110 AND 111, RESPECTIVELY.

weightlifting federation, the Federazione Atletica Italiana (FAI), that Monticelli Obizzi founded in January 1902.

Before 1907, the FAI did not organise official competitions for middleweights, so Gamba was compelled to compete in one class against heavier lifters and among them, very good champions like Scuri, Muggiani, Camillotti, and Ruggeri. It is a pity because he was at his prime from 1903 to 1905, and comparing his achievements to those of lifters of the same weight, the results show that he was the best European athlete. In 1903 he missed the Italian championships because of his academic engagements, and in 1904 he finished runner-up in a controversial contest which took place in Turin on 12 June. The local Turin daily *La Stampa* and the German journal *Illustrierte Athletik Sportzeitung* affirmed that the competition consisted of eight events, but the FAI officially announced that only five of them would count toward the results. Again, *La Stampa* asserted that after the eight exercises, Gamba and the eventual winner, Muggiani from Milan, had totalled the same aggregate of lifted kilos, but the Milanese had been preferred for having a better style. Instead, the official FAI communication referred to five results, and Muggiani won with a higher total.

The one-hand clean and jerk was Gamba's forte and no other European lifter could boast of his record of 82 kg in that specialty. He improved his record in 1905 to 82.20 and then to 84 kg. In that year, turmoil inside the FAI led to the cancellation of the Italian championships. On 2 April Gamba took part in the international contest organised by *L'Education Physique* and jerked 120 kg with two hands in the clean style. Few middleweight lifters in Europe had the same record in the same style. A serious injury obliged Gamba to miss the season in 1906.

In 1907, the FAI introduced the three weight classes in the national contests, keeping a fourth division, the absolute class, free of any weight limit. Finally, Gamba conquered a national title, in the middleweight division, placing runner-up in the absolute. Again in 1908, another academic engagement caused him to miss the national contest. In 1909, the FAI changed the programme and re-proposed a single category for all lifters; in spite of this, Gamba defeated everybody, heavyweights included, snatching 95 kg with two hands. In 1907, Maspoli had lifted the same weight in the French championships in the heavyweight class!

In 1910, the FAI reintroduced the four classes of 1907 and Gamba triumphed in the middleweight and absolute classes. It was the only time a middleweight defeated a heavyweight in Italian history until 1925 when the absolute class became extinct. After two years of inactivity, Gamba came back and won two other Italian middleweight titles in 1913 and 1914. During his eleven competitive seasons, Gamba always performed at a high standard, close to his best records.

A quiet man, venerated by students for his human values, Gamba died in Bellagio on 29 October 1957.

> THE ONE-HAND CLEAN AND JERK WAS GAMBA'S FORTE AND NO OTHER EUROPEAN LIFTER COULD BOAST OF HIS RECORD OF 82 KG IN THAT SPECIALTY.

# The Primordial Rust Belt Workout:
## Chained to Power

### Steven Helmicki
Author of *The Art of the Neck: Training for Distortion* and *Primordial Strength System*

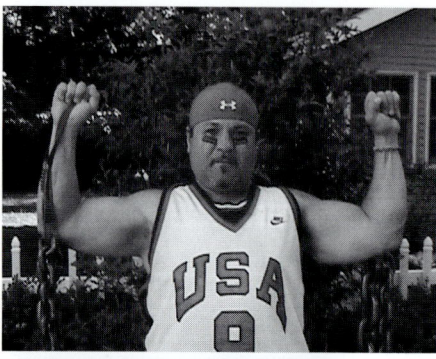

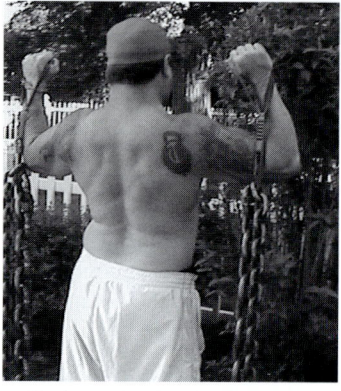

**Chain and Daisy Chain setup.**
Photos courtesy of Steven Helmicki.

*Fundamental tools and philosophies guide us to experience growth at its outer limits.*

Often times the simplest implements can be combined with some good science and economy of time to produce maximized results and still remain tied to the old-school movements. Start with lengths of chain with an IronMind Daisy Chain attached to each, bring along your Headstrap Fit for Hercules and SUPER SQUATS Hip Belt, and you can train anywhere.

The setup for the chains is as follows: The Daisy Chains are looped through the first set of chains. The additional chains slide over the Daisy Chains. The lengths can vary as long as they match on each side (e.g. a 2-foot length on each side, a 3-foot length on each side). You can also vary the sizes of the links. The red loop of the Daisy Chain becomes the handle.

Train three days per week for six weeks. Add one set to each complex per week and watch your explosive power-endurance skyrocket with equipment you can carry in a gym bag wherever you go. Train to win. Period.

> . . . WATCH YOUR EXPLOSIVE POWER–ENDURANCE SKYROCKET WITH EQUIPMENT YOU CAN CARRY IN A GYM BAG . . .

## Chain workout – 3 days per week x 6 weeks

**Day 1**

- Chain squat (2 sets of chain) x 4
- Chain squat (4 sets of chain) x 4
  Repeat 3 times non-stop

Hydration

- Chain military press (2 sets of chain) x 4
- Chain squat (4 sets of chain) x 4
  Repeat 3 times non-stop

Hydration

- Chain curls (2 sets of chain) x 4
- Chain squat (4 sets of chain) x 4
  Repeat 3 times non-stop

Hydration

- Chain triceps extension, standing (2 sets of chain) x 4
- Chain squat (4 sets of chain) x 4
  Repeat 3 times non-stop

Hydration

- Chain neck harness extension/flexion (2 sets of chain) x 4
- Chain squat (4 sets of chain) x 4
  Repeat 3 times non-stop

**Day 2**

- Chain squat (3 sets of chain) x 2
- Chain squats (6 sets of chain) x 2
  Repeat 2 times non-stop

Hydration

- Chain incline presses (2 sets of chain) x 4
- Chain incline bench (4 sets of chain) x 4
  Repeat 3 times non-stop

Hydration

- Chain chin-ups (2 sets of chain) x 2
- Chain chin-ups (4 sets of chain) x 2
  Repeat 3 times non-stop

Hydration

- Chain shrugs (3 sets of chain) x 5
- Chain shrugs (6 sets of chain) x 5
  Repeat 2 times non-stop

Hydration

- Chain sit-ups (2 sets of chain) x 5
- Chain sit-ups (4 sets of chain) x 5
- Repeat 2 times non-stop

Hydration

Neck harness with 1 set of chain x 30 reps extension/flexion

**Day 3**

- Chain stiff-legged deadlifts (2 sets of chain) x 3
- Chain stiff-legged deadlifts (4 sets of chain) x 3
  Repeat 3 times non-stop

Hydration

- Chain bent-over rows (2 sets of chain) x 5
- Chain bent-over rows (4 sets of chain) x 5
  Repeat 3 times non-stop

Hydration

- Chain bench press (3 sets of chain) x 4
- Chain bench press (6 sets of chain) x 4
  Repeat 2 times non-stop

Hydration

- Chain curls (2 sets of chain) x 25 reps

Hydration

Neck harness (3 sets of chain) x 15 reps flexion/extension

## Getting Things Straight, Part II:
# Hardball Training

**Dr. Ken E. Leistner**
Chiropractor

"**G**etting Things Straight, Part I: 'Core' Principles" in the June 2010 issue of MILO seemed to be a revelation to some readers; yet from my perspective, it was no more than a recounting of some basic facts steeped in logic and common sense. There are some dyed-in-the-wool, enthusiastic young trainees who do, or at least did, believe that picking up a basic anatomical text would reveal which specific muscles were one's "core." Those who know me understand that I am just not the kind of person to go intellectual and even begin a conversation about getting to one's core and then going off on a discourse about the soul of man or the philosophical beliefs tied to one's inner organs, so maintaining the pathway started in Part I, let us get serious about productive training.

Anyone's body, his physical "plant," his basic physiology, seeks homeostasis. This big word just means that wherever your bodily functions happen to be for a period of time is the place your body wants to remain. For example, if your normal bodyweight hovers between 188 and 190 lb., you are going to have to work a bit to move it out of its comfort zone. If you can squat 300 x 5, you are going to have to fight a lot and endure some discomfort to move that squat poundage up to 325 x 5. For those of us who have made significant or wholesale alterations in our physiques or strength levels, we know there are reasons that they just don't come easily. The media would have you believe otherwise.

If one is gainfully employed and has more or less normal 8 to 5 or 9 to 5 work hours, he misses some of the most unpleasant television ever dreamed of. In our facility, we keep a television on all day and evening to allow those using the cardio equipment to warm up, do cardiac-related rehabilitation, or cool down with something to look at to relieve the boredom of maintaining one's pulse rate within appropriate parameters for a 20- to 40-minute period while indoors. It has always been my belief that it is more effective and more enjoyable to chase after something, like a ball, or otherwise have constant movement for an extended time if outdoors. However, when physiological monitoring is necessary and/or the weather will not allow outdoor activity, its best to use a treadmill, stationary bicycle, elliptical machine, or anything that allows for steady-state activity.

ESPN and related sports shows are popular with most of our athletes, but we claim a segment of individuals who watch the junk, reality-type television shows that can produce howls of laughter, even knowing that "reality shows" are for the most part very carefully scripted by producers, directors, and a

> IF YOU CAN SQUAT 300 x 5, YOU ARE GOING TO HAVE TO FIGHT A LOT AND ENDURE SOME DISCOMFORT TO MOVE THAT SQUAT POUNDAGE UP TO 325 x 5.

creative team that gets paid a great deal of money to keep the public's interest.

In the early 1980s, I had the distinction of having appeared on a number of nationally broadcast daytime television shows, including the show hosted by my patient at the time, Regis Philbin (who was and I am sure remains, a very "regular" person off the set, an enlightened sports fan, and a very funny guy). As was carefully explained to me as I was prepped for the *Hour Magazine* show, one of the first of the mainstream late morning talk-cum-entertainment programs, I had to speak to the viewing audience and I had to remember that this audience was predominantly twenty-one- to thirty-five-year-old females with one to three children. As the producer said to me, "You are addressing a twenty-two-year-old stay-at-home housewife with two children in Iowa." I indicated that I got it and that I would walk across the stage and not ambulate from one point to another. This won approving smiles from all.

The current state of television has degenerated significantly as noted by one of my long-time trainees, a New York City court officer who appears on one of the very popular judge shows as the court officer. His comment, comparing my caustic commentary about the state of the culture was, "Yes, but now the audience, at least for my show, is the same housewife who probably isn't married and lives in a trailer park somewhere in Kentucky." The point? The commercials for all of these programs are selling a vast array of things one needs to use or do in order to lose body fat, get thinner, firm the triceps and biceps, build the strength and hard-as-a-rock appearance of the abs and core, and of course, perform better sexually as doing all of the above is supposed to contribute to this enhanced performance.

I have yet to see or hear any commercial boost the benefits of doing barbell squats, presses, deadlifts, or pulls from the floor. If one truly wants to be harder, one has to build muscle tissue. If a female or male wishes to have better shape and tone, he or she must lift weights in a progressive manner in order to stimulate muscle tissue growth because it is the developed muscle that gives the body shape and form over and above what one is born with. So-called core strength, any amount of strength, is not developed by doing a shaking motion with a 2.5-lb. dumbbell with some sort of spring apparatus tucked into the handle.

> I HAVE YET TO SEE OR HEAR ANY COMMERCIAL BOOST THE BENEFITS OF DOING BARBELL SQUATS, PRESSES, DEADLIFTS, OR PULLS FROM THE FLOOR.

There is nothing like seeing a photo of a fitness model who has been filmed while in top shape juxtaposed with a photo taken after paying him to eat and drink himself out of shape for a month or two; these photos are then flipped so that the true "after" shot of the sort-of-in-shape-but-sagging midsection now becomes the "before" photo, with the implication or outright assertion that the item being advertised was responsible for the dramatic turnaround that resulted in cut-up, almost physique-contest condition. Strength increases that allow for true athletic success come from hard, consistent work pulling barbells, stones, or other implements off of the floor, yet I have not seen an advertisement for a set of lifting stones while watching NFL football.

Common sense, when applied to one's physiology, would surely indicate that one has to train very hard to get meaningful results and that to become truly strong, one needs the modalities to do it. Pushing 5-, 10-, or 20-lb. weights on any type of machine is not going to make anyone very strong. Standing on an inflated ball, even if balancing on one foot, is not going to allow for the use of weights significant enough to stimulate changes in anyone's body unless he is recovering from an illness or long-term physical inertia. Yet, I am sure that if one examined the income made from barbells, dumbbells, stones, and kettlebells, it would be a pittance compared to that of even one of the core, ab, or total-body machines anyone can buy via mail order. The public has to be a lot smarter or otherwise be willing to admit it will remain weak, overweight, overfat, and yes, needing more sexual enhancement!

Basic hardball training on a few exercises that can be done at home as well as in a commercial gym or institutional weightroom is all that any man or woman needs to truly transform his or her muscular system.

> THE PUBLIC HAS TO BE A LOT SMARTER OR OTHERWISE BE WILLING TO ADMIT IT WILL REMAIN WEAK, OVERWEIGHT, OVERFAT, AND YES, NEEDING MORE SEXUAL ENHANCEMENT!

Instead of the Ab-Envy machine, Core Controller, and I Am Sexier Now Than I Was Yesterday Enhancer, try this at home for six weeks:

**Day 1**

| | |
|---|---|
| Dumbbell press | warm up x 6; work sets 1 x 12; 1 x 6 |
| Dumbbell row | 1 x 12; 1 x 6 |
| Dumbbell deadlift | 1 x 15; 1 x 6 |
| Barbell press | 1 x 8; 1 x 5 |
| Barbell row | 1 x 8; 1 x 5 |
| Barbell deadlift | 1 x 8; 1 x 5 |

Sit-ups 1 x 20, as with any other movement, progressively add resistance

**Day 2**

| | |
|---|---|
| Bench press | warm up x 8; work sets 1 x 12; 1 x 6 |
| Chin-up (or negative chin-ups) | 1 set of 6 reps, progressively until strong enough to add reps until 2 x 10 and then when capable of doing so, progressively add resistance |
| Close-grip push-up | 1 x max reps done slowly |
| Barbell curl | 1 x 12; 1 x 6 |
| Barbell squat | warm up x 10; work sets 1 x 25; 1 x 15 |

Sit-ups as per Day 1

# John Godina:
## World-Class Throwing Drug-Free

### Thom Van Vleck

Over the years, I have participated in and enjoyed all types of strength sports, from Olympic lifting and powerlifting to all-round lifting and strongman. I have also enjoyed throwing, from track and field events to Scottish Highland Games athletics. During that time, I have decorated my gym, the Jackson Weightlifting Club, with pictures of my favorite athletes. Watching and participating in these strength events has offered me the chance to meet many of the people in the photos, and whenever I do, I have a lot of questions. I just seem to have a drive to acquire every little morsel of knowledge I can find on strength sports.

Recently, work took to me the Phoenix, Arizona area, and I immediately tried to think of whom I could visit in Arizona to expand my strength training knowledge. I was talking this over with John Gallagher, two-time Highland Games stone put world champion who knows a thing or two about throwing, and he said, "If you are going to Arizona and you want to learn more about explosive strength, there's only one guy you want to visit, John Godina." Gallagher knows I'm also big on drug-free training. I planned my trip and made arrangements to visit John Godina.

Godina only recently retired after a pretty amazing career. He won the world championships in the shot put outdoors in 1995, just months after winning NCAA titles in both the shot and discus and setting a record of 22.0 m, which remains unbroken after 15 years. He was the world champion again in 1997 and 2001, and he also won an indoor world title in 2001. Three times an Olympian (1996, 2000, 2004) and twice an Olympic medalist in the shot put, he won silver in the 1996 Olympics and bronze in 2000.

John's prowess was not just in the shot put. He was also a two-time U.S. discus champion and in 1996 became the first American in 72 years to make the U.S. Olympic team in both the shot and discus. His six appearances at the world championships (outdoors) tie him for the most by an American male thrower. Godina was also a two-time Jesse Owens award winner as the top male track-and-field athlete in the U.S.

In the shot put, John has a personal best of 22.20 m (72' 10") set in 2005 and in the discus, 69.91 m (229' 4") set in 1998.

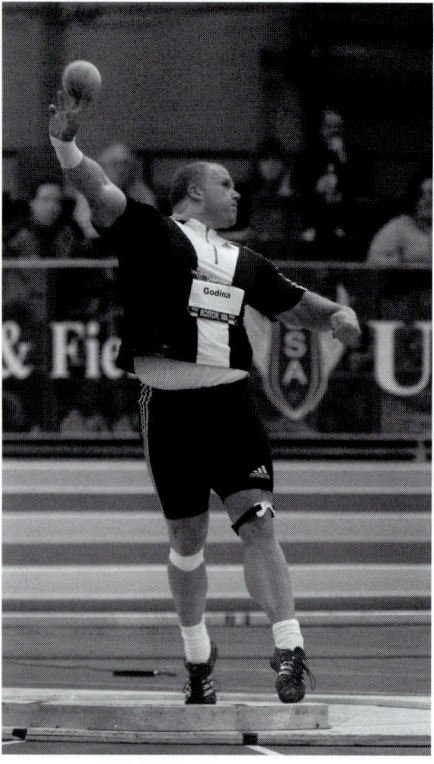

**John Godina in the shot put.**
Victor Sailer photo.

John listed his career highlights in this order:

1. The 1995 NCAA Championships where he threw 22.00 m in the shot put. John told me, "It changed my whole career." He is proud of the fact that the throw was not only a record then but is still the record today. I noted that the only real trophy that decorated his office was the toe board from that championships. No medals, no plaques . . . just the toe board!

2. In the 1998 season John went over 21.00 m in every event and didn't lose in the shot put all year while also doing well in the discus (it was also the year he hit his lifetime PR).

3. In 2001 John was undefeated until the Goodwill Games, winning the indoor and outdoor world championships.

John has the respect of the greats. Here is what Al Feuerbach had to say about Godina: "John Godina makes me feel proud to be called a thrower. He is intelligent and respectful, and is a master technician. There were the throwers like Brian Oldfield, who was like a wild man, and throwers like Randy Matson, who was so technically and physically talented that he didn't have to say a single thing to gain your respect and awe. I guess in a way John Godina is a bit of a combination of those different types of great throwers. He had to work for it and he did. He became great at more than one event on the world stage and all the while he portrayed an image of being humble. That makes someone colorful in my book!"

> "HE BECAME GREAT AT MORE THAN ONE EVENT ON THE WORLD STAGE AND ALL THE WHILE HE PORTRAYED AN IMAGE OF BEING HUMBLE. THAT MAKES SOMEONE COLORFUL IN MY BOOK!"

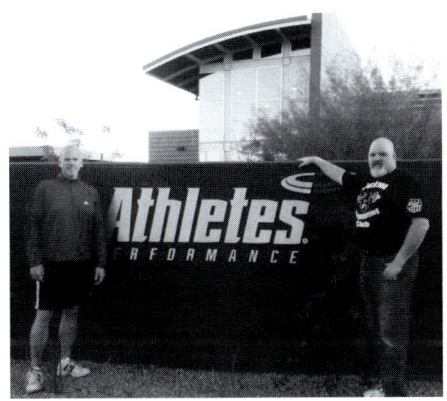

**Thom Van Vleck (r.) and John Godina (l.) in front of the World Throws Center.**
Courtesy of Thom Van Vleck.

I arranged to meet with John at Athlete's Performance where he runs the John Godina World Throws Center. This is an amazing facility geared toward the elite athlete, covering every facet of training from exercise to diet, physical therapy, and more. While I was visiting with John, he was training Om Prakash Karahana Singh (or O. P. for short . . . and I can understand why!). John explained the high-tech approach they take at Athlete's Performance, showing me O. P.'s 43-week training routine. He clicked buttons which translated the lifting and throwing into graphs denoting a progression toward a peak. The detail was amazing. As we talked, John revealed what a task master he could be, exhorting O. P. to work harder from rep to rep and lift to lift.

John told me that Athlete's Performance was started by Mark Verstegan and that his World Throws Center was a part of the facility. I had come the week after they had had some 25 potential NFL draftees on site preparing for the NFL Combine. He said they train a lot of top athletes from the NFL, NBA, NHL, and MLB as well as national and world caliber athletes from other sports. This facility is something special, and John said he thinks it's the best in the world of its kind. It was hard to miss the endless autographed jerseys that lined the walls of the facility, and every corner brought a new dimension to the services they offer. John explained that they are looking to expand their facilities to accommodate a throwing ring on site (they currently have to take throwers elsewhere to practice) and other improvements geared just to throwers. He seems to have embraced his new role as a coach and is approaching it with the same drive he did as a thrower.

Just recently Godina paired with Ryan Vierra (five-time pro Highland Games world champion) to hold a Highland Games throwing seminar at the World Throws Center. Ryan was a thrower at California State University, Northridge (CSUN), and he and Godina threw against each other during the 1991 and 1992 seasons, becoming friends along the way. Ryan's coach at CSUN, John Frazier, had come from UCLA where John Godina was then throwing and as a result, Ryan and John had very similar training philosophies. Over the years they kept in touch and when the athletic director of the Arizona Highland Games, Ryan Seckman, suggested they host a seminar focusing on the heavy events, they were all for it.

Godina seemed very enthusiastic as he talked about training Highland Games athletes, and stated that he really admired the top throwers in that sport. He said he knows how difficult it is to master two throwing events at the same time, let alone all those required

> HE JUST SHOOK HIS HEAD AT THE THOUGHT OF THROWING A 56-LB. WEIGHT-FOR-DISTANCE AND ASKED, "HOW CAN ANYONE THROW THAT THING?"

to be a top Highland Games pro. He just shook his head at the thought of throwing a 56-lb. weight-for-distance and asked, "How can anyone throw that thing?" Godina is excited about the prospect of doing more work with Scottish Highland Games athletes in the future.

Dave Brown, a top Highland Games pro heavy and a world record-holder in the 56-lb. weight-over-bar at 20' 1", attended that seminar. He told me that he had been to "nearly a hundred clinics . . . I wouldn't call this a clinic at all . . . call it a mega-clinic." Dave went on to say, "If you wanted to go somewhere that would show some improvement and get a pat on the back for the weekend and only add a few feet to an event, then this is not the place for you. Instead, if you desire not just to throw better, but also to learn how to throw at the peak of your mechanics and mental aptitude, this instruction is miles ahead of anything else you've probably seen and you would want to make sure the video camera has plenty of battery."

I asked John whom he looked up to or admired. He said, "I was never really one to put someone on a pedestal but I owe a lot to Mac Wilkins and if I had to pick an athlete I most admired, it would be Al Oerter based on his accomplishments." John stated that he was helped most by Art Venegas and a 14-year coaching relationship that started at UCLA, and that Art had the greatest impact on his career.

> JOHN TOLD ME THAT HE WAS NEVER MUCH INTO MEDIUM OR LIGHT DAYS, "WHEN YOU GO, YOU GO AND WHEN YOU REST, YOU REST."

We talked a great deal about training. John told me that he was never much into medium or light days, "When you go, you go and when you rest, you rest." He said his training has changed as he ages. For example, he initially squatted once a week, then once every 10 days, then once every 14 days, and finally about twice a month or less. John said he always wanted to feel rested and ready to go and that led to the increased periods of recuperation as he got older.

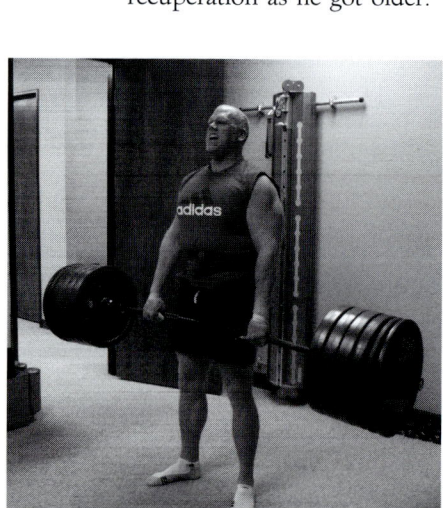

**Recent unpublished photo of John Godina deadlifting.**
Courtesy of John Godina.

On training, John told me, "I rarely missed lifting a weight in training because to me, failure is not when you miss a weight, but when technique breaks down, which always happens

**56 MILO** | September 2010, Vol. 18, No. 2

first." He sees training as much more mental than physical, calling it an "education of the mind." He then told me, "You can do a lot more than you think you can." John said, "You need to have an intelligent plan or you will get hurt. When you get hurt, you begin to think you can't, and when you think you can't, then you won't."

We then got into the subject of performance-enhancing drugs in sports. One of the main reasons I wanted to talk to Godina was the fact that I had heard he was a drug-free thrower. When I asked Ryan Vierra what he thought of Godina, the first thing he mentioned was, "[Godina is the] . . . best clean shot putter of all time." Sean Betz, 2008 pro Highland Games world champion and a proponent of being drug-free, also made this same statement as the one thing that defined Godina above all others.

Godina is not only drug-free, but he is a vocal advocate about it. He told me, "People who use [drugs] are cowards because they are afraid to find out if they are the best without it. There can be only one, so either work hard to be that one or accept that you aren't." As we continued to talk about training, John stated, "Take the time to develop real strength and don't take a short cut with drugs. Sure, drugs will make you stronger and faster, but strength doesn't go away if it comes legitimately in the first place."

When I brought up with Sean Betz that I was working on a story about John Godina, I never intended to ask him for a quote, but Sean told me he had admired John for a long time—and not just his stance on performance-enhancing drugs. Sean grew up less than an hour away from where John grew up and recalled reading a story about him when Sean was a sophomore in high school: "I remember hearing about him being a football legend in high school and he could have pretty much played anywhere, but he chose to throw instead." He recalled John not only being very strong but being fast as well, running a 4.6-second 40-yard dash. It is amazing the impact people can have on others.

I asked Godina about football and he stated that he was offered many scholarships and could have easily gone in that direction. When asked why he didn't, John said, "I didn't like practice, and training for football was listening to coaches and following their plan . . . but training for throwing was a puzzle you put together yourself." I think most strength sports athletes could identify with that statement. I know I did.

> "People who use [drugs] are cowards because they are afraid to find out if they are the best without it."

Finally, Ryan Vierra told me that he was most impressed with "John's throwing *and* his character and personality. His attention to detail . . . the man conducts every aspect of his life in a professional manner." After visiting with John Godina, I felt the same way. I hope he does another Highland Games clinic with Vierra and if he does, I will be there. I also appreciate his stance on performance-enhancing drugs and not being afraid to say it. Sure, it takes talent to be a great athlete, but it also takes heart and intelligence, and John Godina has all three. M

## Carnivores and Cancer:
# Where's the Beef?

### Steve Milloy
JunkScience.com

If you're a *MILO* reader, you probably eat meat and dairy products—a lot. Both are great sources of protein and other essential nutrients. But you may also have heard that consumption of animal protein causes or increases the risk of a variety of health problems, including diseases like cancer and heart disease.

You'll hear these claims from many dieticians, physicians, public health advocates, medical researchers, and organizations like the American Cancer Society and the federal government's National Cancer Institute. But you'll hear denials of these claims from other scientists and physicians, and business associations like the National Cattleman's Beef Association and the American Meat Institute.

### So who is right and how can you tell?

It's easy for me to make the call since I am a trained biostatistician and have been chronicling these and many other science and public health controversies for more than 14 years at my web site JunkScience.com, which should be a big hint as to where I will come out on the question Is meat bad for you? At JunkScience.com, we take no prisoners when it comes to baseless fearmongering, especially when it is driven by social, political and other, often hidden, agendas.

That said, it is impossible to completely debunk all the claims and scares about meat and dairy consumption in a single *MILO* article. Many different types and quantities of meat and dairy consumption have allegedly been linked with a multitude of ailments in a variety of study types. There is simply not enough space here to address them all, but to get what is sure to be a hot debate rolling, I've decided to focus on a two animal protein scares as a start to provide *MILO* readers with the tools for self-defense against junk science.

### Rats aren't little people

A book entitled *The China Study* seems to be the basis for the current rumor that milk protein (casein) increases cancer risk. According to the book, laboratory rats were initially dosed with aflatoxin, a potent cancer-causing substance, and then fed either high (20%)

> THE FIRST RULE IN DEBUNKING JUNK SCIENCE WHEN DEALING WITH ANIMAL STUDIES IS THIS: MICE (AND RATS) ARE NOT LITTLE PEOPLE.

or low (5%) casein diets for twelve weeks. The rats were then sacrificed and examined for liver foci development—clusters of cells that can be a precursor to cancer. The researcher, who is also the co-author of the book, reported that the rats on the high-protein diet had more liver foci than rats on the low-protein diet. If *The China Study* has put you off milk, ask yourself this, Am I a poisoned rat?

The first rule in debunking junk science when dealing with animal studies is this: mice (and rats) are not little people. This is especially true of the sort of lab rats used in this particular study. They were specially bred to be predisposed to cancer, so prone in fact that the biggest cancer risk in their two-year long lives was the amount of food they ate—the more they ate, the more cancer they tended to develop. It's quite possible (if not likely) that the explanation for the increased liver foci observed in the rats that ate the high-protein diet is that the high-protein diet tasted better and they ate more. But then we're really getting ahead of ourselves here since most foci don't develop into tumors and not all tumors are cancerous. And let's not forget that these animals were given a high dose of a potent carcinogen to get the liver foci ball rolling in the first place. Neither these rats nor what happened to them is relevant to your physiology or your consumption of casein-containing dairy products and protein supplements.

The fact that the book's author spends so much time describing rat studies should also tell you something else. He can't point to credible studies of humans that implicate casein in the development of cancer.

But what would you do if he did?

### Epidemiology is statistics, not science

It wasn't hard to locate such a scare involving a study of humans. I did a Google news search on "meat and cancer" on March 27, 2010 and came up with a headline that read "Red Meat, Obesity Raise the Risk of Colon Cancer." The article reported that "a team from the division of Cancer Epidemiology and Genetics at the U.S. National Cancer Institute . . . reviewed a cohort of 300,000 men and women . . . [and concluded in the March 15, 2010 issue of *Cancer Research* that] . . . those who ate the most red and processed meat showed a significantly higher risk of developing colorectal cancer than those . . . who consumed the least amount of meat."

> THE AVERAGE PERSON—EVEN THE AVERAGE PHYSICIAN—READING THE ARTICLE IS LIKELY GOING TO LOOK AT HIS CHEESEBURGER SKEPTICALLY AND THINK TWICE BEFORE SWALLOWING.

The average person—even the average physician—reading the article is likely going to look at his cheeseburger skeptically and think twice before swallowing. Consider the article's salient points: *Government* scientists studied *300,000 people* and reported in a *prestigious-sounding medical journal* that eating meat is putting you at risk of the *second leading cause of cancer deaths* in the western world. What can you do in the face of such apparent authority but trash your cheeseburger in favor of a soy burger—after all, it is said, some really do taste like meat.

But I'm not giving up cheeseburgers and here's why.

The primary results from this study are as follows: (1) there was 24% more colorectal cancer among those who ate the most red meat as compared to those who ate the least; and (2) there was 16% more colorectal cancer among those who ate the most processed meat as compared to those who ate the least. While the study authors observed in their study that these increases are merely statistical associations or correlations, the news article reported them as definite increases in risk.

The first thing to realize is that statistical correlation is not the same as causation or cause-in-fact. To understand the difference consider that urban areas have comparatively more traffic and crime than rural areas. More traffic congestion correlates with higher crime rates. That said, traffic doesn't cause crime.

Back to our study. Accepting the study results at face value, the authors have reported more cancer among those who ate more meat. That may very well be the case among these particular study subjects, but it doesn't mean that eating meat has anything to do with the observed cases of cancer.

> BUT I'M NOT GIVING UP CHEESEBURGERS AND HERE'S WHY.

Epidemiologists (researchers who study the patterns of disease among populations) have a rule of thumb for interpreting the sort of statistical association and correlations reported in the study; it is this: "In epidemiologic research, [increases in risk of less than 100%] are considered small and usually difficult to interpret. Such increases may be due to chance, statistical bias or effects of confounding factors that are sometimes not evident."

So while the increases in risk in our study (24% and 16%) may seem large, they are actually too small for the researchers to have reliably detected through standard epidemiologic techniques. But what about those expert government researchers who studied 300,000 people and reported their results in a peer-reviewed journal? What about them? Scientific conclusions depend on the intrinsic *quality* of data and analysis, not the *quantity* of data or preconceptions about who did the analysis.

The basic problem with epidemiologic studies (especially when it comes to weak correlations involving common diseases like colorectal cancer) is that the quality of the data used in the statistical analyses tends to, well, suck.

First, no one really knows how much meat (or anything else) the study subjects actually consumed. Study subjects were asked to recall what and how much they ate on one day in 1995. That response was then assumed to be their meat consumption every day for the next seven years. Whoever had a 20-ounce Porterhouse steak the day of the survey is assumed to have consumed that same steak every day for the seven years of the study. Whoever had a chicken sandwich instead of a burger that day is assumed to have not eaten meat for the duration of the study. Then there's the problem of people who forgot what they ate or over- or under-reported how much they ate. There is no magical statistical wand that may be waved to make these deficiencies go away.

Next, the data are woefully incomplete, particularly with respect to so-called confounding risk factors for colorectal cancer.

Although no one knows what causes colorectal cancer (and lack of fiber is not a risk factor, but that's a story for another day), it is thought that one's risk may be affected by age (perhaps the greatest risk factor of all for cancer generally), family history of cancer (indicating a genetic predisposition to cancer), race (African-Americans and Ashkenazi Jews seems to experience higher rates of colorectal cancer), heavy smoking and drinking, and physical inactivity, to name just a few factors that have been identified.

In the study we're considering, the only confounding risk factors considered were age, socio-economic status (poor people tend to be less healthy), smoking and caloric intake. This is hardly a comprehensive consideration of risk factors.

Keep in mind that not one of these 300,000 study subjects was individually examined by any sort of expert and not one of the 2,719 cases of colorectal cancer was biologically or medically determined to have been caused by meat consumption. This study is entirely statistical in nature—and you know what they say about statistics and the people who use them.

For my money, this study is nothing short of GIGO—garbage in, garbage out.

But didn't *government* scientists do the research? If the study is so bad, then how did it get past peer review to be published in what seems to be a reputable journal?

What you have to remember is that scientists are not some higher form of life than you. As is true with people and professionals from all walks of life, there are the good and the bad, the competent and the incompetent, and the ethical and the unethical.

Like all organizations, the government is made up of and led by all sorts of the aforementioned people. Scientists and government agencies often have agendas that they try to advance through "scientific research." When you get down to it, the National Cancer Institute is just another government agency with its own politics and budget needs. You invest organizations with more authority than they merit at your own risk.

The main author of the study we've been considering is a vegetarian who has used her post at the National Cancer Institute to advance the anti-meat agenda for more than a decade. She has published numerous studies all claiming to link meat-eating with cancer. Though all her studies suffer from the same fatal flaws that have been mentioned here, she succeeds in scaring people time after time because a gullible and sensationalist mainstream media is

> THE MEDIA IS A VERY IMPORTANT TOOL OF THE JUNK SCIENCE CROWD.

always looking to publish scary news stories. The media is a very important tool of the junk science crowd.

Finally, keep in mind that humans evolved as meat-eaters. It is unlikely that man evolved to consume an inherently self-destructive diet. So-called "natural" food stores may push a vegetarian or grain-based diet, but man is naturally a meat-eater. Just look at your front teeth—they are designed to tear at flesh. Compare your sharp teeth with those of an herbivore like a cow.

A grain-based diet only evolved recently with the advent of organized agriculture production (about 10,000 years ago). None of this is to knock a vegetarian diet, but it is merely a food or lifestyle preference, not a recipe for better health or athletic performance—and I challenge anyone to show me a specific piece of research that proves the contrary.

So that's a window into the world of debunking junk science-fueled health scares. There is much more that can and needs to be said to debunk the numerous meat and dairy scares, but this has been a start. **M**

# The Country Mile

## John Brookfield

*Author of* Mastery of Hand Strength, Revised Edition, The Grip Master's Manual, Training with Cables for Strength, *and* Dexterity Ball Training for Hands

In this article we will look at a results-producing workout that will give you a full-body workout while covering distance at the same time. You will be using one of the best natural training objects around, the stone. As I have mentioned in the past, I have found that by simply carrying a stone you get one of the best strength and endurance workouts under the sun. In fact, you work your entire body in a world-class functional way while you are using and enhancing your cardiovascular system at the same time. The object of this workout is to lift a good-sized stone and hold it against your chest as you walk.

I like to call this workout the Country Mile because you will be carrying your stone for a full mile. To get the full benefit from the Country Mile workout, the stone will be carried against your chest instead of on your shoulder. This way, you are totally engaged and fighting to keep yourself from bending forward as you walk. You will need a good-sized stone for this workout, but be sure that your stone is not so heavy that you can't carry it safely as you walk.

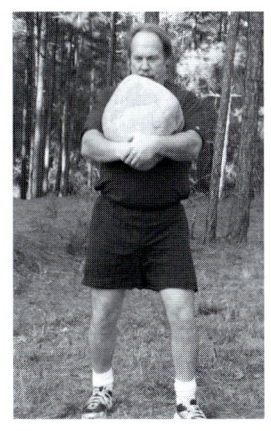

**Walking the Country Mile.**
Photo courtesy of John Brookfield.

For the Country Mile workout I like to carry a stone weighing anywhere from 100 lb. all the way up to 160 lb., depending on the terrain and on how fast I want to cover the distance. It is best to have a stone that is not too sharp: a smooth, creek-type stone will work best so that you can concentrate on the walking and not be sidetracked by the abrasiveness of the stone.

I have been asked quite often whether a heavy barbell plate, like a 100-pounder, would work just as well as the stone for this exercise. The answer to this is no—the heavy plate will not be nearly so effective. You can carry one if you want and it will give you a workout, but because it is so flat, you will be holding it right up against your chest. On the other hand, the stone, being much larger and thicker, will be protruding in front of you and will force your core and your entire body to work harder and remain stabilized as you walk carrying the stone. This effect, of course, is based on the same idea that the farther a weight is out in front of you, the harder it is to lift.

Once you have chosen your stone, you need to choose your mile—your walking route. You will want to mark off a full mile for the Country Mile workout.

I suggest doing a half mile one way and a half mile back for the full mile. If you live in an area that is not user-friendly for carrying a stone a half mile and back, you can either take a short drive with your stone to a better spot or, if need be, you can go up and down your driveway the number of times it takes to go a full mile.

You can either carry a watch in your pocket or you can mark the time when you start and again when you finish if you are starting and finishing in the same place. You may have noticed I said that you will want to carry the watch in your pocket. If it is on your wrist, you will probably break it or scuff it up, or it will scrape your wrist when pressed by the stone. Once you have chosen your spot and are ready to mark your time, you are ready for the Country Mile.

Lift the stone and secure it against your chest as you start walking your route. Be sure to keep your body upright and watch your footing as you walk forward carrying the stone. Keep moving at a slow and steady pace, striving to keep the stone against your chest and not set it down.

Go as far as you can before stopping and then set it down and take a break, keeping it as short as possible. Once you have recovered slightly, pick up the stone again and take off carrying the stone against your chest. Go as far as you can again and then stop and set the stone down for another short break. As you can see, the object of the Country Mile workout is to carry the stone for the entire mile, keeping up as good a pace as possible. Once you get to the halfway spot a half mile out, turn around and carry the stone back the other half mile to the starting spot. Your other goal, in addition to carrying the stone a mile, is to put the stone down as few times as possible during the Country Mile workout.

As you improve you will have to put the stone down less frequently during the walk, which will of course make your time faster. Strive to carry the stone farther and farther each workout until you get to where you hardly have to set it down at all. Of course this will depend on how heavy and awkward your stone is. Remember that you are competing against yourself and when your time gets better, you are the winner. As you improve and can go the entire time with setting the stone down only a few times or not at all, you can move up to a heavier stone. With a heavier stone, of course, you use the same format and carry the stone for the Country Mile, setting it down as few times as possible.

The next level of difficulty on the Country Mile workout gets quite interesting to say the least. You will be carrying a stone a mile against your chest in the same fashion; however, this time when you have to stop and put the stone down, instead of resting you will be doing push-ups. Do as many push-ups as you can until you feel the fatigue in your upper body. As soon as you feel fatigued from the push-ups, pick up the stone, hold it against your chest, and start walking again. Go as far as possible until you have to put the stone down again. Once you set it down there is no rest and you do the push-ups again until you are fatigued. Pick up the stone and carry it as far as possible, set it down, and do the push-ups. Continue doing the combination of carrying the stone as far as possible and then doing the push-ups until you have covered the entire mile.

After you put the stone down and finish the push-ups the first time, you may find yourself doing shorter and shorter stone carries and fewer repetitions on the push-ups. This is normal, but push yourself to keep going and each workout will get a bit better—your endurance will improve and you will be carrying the stone farther each time and recovering more quickly after doing the push-ups.

You may find the Country Mile workout difficult, to say the least; however, it is what is needed to develop your strength and endurance and to move to a higher level of physical and mental conditioning that will transfer into anything you do. It is a true test of your physical conditioning and mental fortitude: you will need to stay focused on your destination instead of looking at the obstacles and thinking about how you feel, if you want to succeed. This workout brings a whole new meaning to the term a country mile. **M**

> REMEMBER THAT YOU ARE COMPETING AGAINST YOURSELF AND WHEN YOUR TIME GETS BETTER, YOU ARE THE WINNER.

> . . . YOU WILL NEED TO STAY FOCUSED ON YOUR DESTINATION INSTEAD OF LOOKING AT THE OBSTACLES AND THINKING ABOUT HOW YOU FEEL, IF YOU WANT TO SUCCEED.

# Running for His Life

### Keith Wassung

Joe Stewart was the epitome of health and fitness. His powerful physique bore witness to his many years of heavy barbell training. A successful real estate agent and the father of three boys, Joe was often mistaken for a man who was ten years younger than his actual forty-six years. He had always been a standout athlete, dominating Little League and Pee Wee football as a youth, and he followed that up with All-State honors in football and track in high school. A full-ride football scholarship to Georgia Tech was short-lived as Joe experienced a career-ending knee injury during his sophomore year. He spent eight months in the school weightroom attempting to rehabilitate it, but was never able to fully recover. He then turned his attention to academics and ended up graduating with high honors and obtaining a business degree. To fill the athletic void, Joe turned to regular barbell training. He had already engaged in some strength training but mostly as an adjunct to football and track. Lifting quickly became his primary focus. By the time he received his MBA, Joe was regularly winning area powerlifting events.

Joe was recruited out of graduate school by a Fortune 500 company and relocated from Georgia to Pensacola, Florida to begin work. Though Joe was earning an impressive income, he quickly grew tired of the corporate grind. While playing golf with some friends, he was introduced to one of the top real estate agents in western Florida. He convinced Joe to leave the corporate job and enter the real estate business. Joe did so and was a natural sales agent. His business grew, as did his family. The hours were still long but very enjoyable. He always managed to find time to continue his workouts. He had had seen far too many middle-aged men who were overweight, unhealthy, and out of shape and he vowed that he would never be one of them. His clients and colleagues often asked him for exercise and diet advice and Joe was more than happy to oblige.

> To fill the athletic void, Joe turned to regular barbell training.

While sitting as his desk one afternoon, a woman from the legal department knocked on his door and asked Joe for a property listing that he had borrowed the day before. She noticed his workout bag on the floor and mentioned that she wished she could start an exercise program of her own. She and Joe talked about it for a few minutes and Joe offered some advice and encouragement to her. She thanked him both for the report and the advice and left his office.

Joe Stewart was the epitome of health and fitness. But he held a deep, dark secret about his health, a secret that only he knew and one that he had kept carefully guarded for the past few

---

**Joe Stewart was the epitome of health and fitness. But he held a deep, dark secret about his health . . .**

years. Joe only gave the appearance of health and fitness; he was actually in horrible shape.

After entering the workplace, Joe had continued an intense conditioning program along with his strength training. But as his business and family grew, he had less and less time for workouts and that time was spent almost exclusively lifting weights. By the time he was in his mid-thirties Joe was doing virtually nothing other than strength training. He would occasionally engage in pick-up games of basketball and touch football and there appeared to be little or no drop-off in his conditioning. He also knew that he could start a conditioning program anytime he wanted to and he could be back in top shape in a month or two. He planned to focus more on conditioning when he turned forty. Forty came and went and Joe continued pounding the heavy iron, often out-squatting men half his age by hundreds of pounds.

The downturn in the economy forced Joe to work longer and harder than he had in many years. Often it was hard to get anyone interested in real estate, but he persisted. He would frequently eat on the run, typically fast food, in an effort to restore his business. He began sleeping less and missing workouts. He also put on 10 to 15 unwanted pounds, which were barely noticeable to anyone other than Joe and his wife, Marie. His energy and vitality begin to deteriorate, and Joe began feeling his age. He still looked fit and strong on the outside, but internally he felt terrible.

Two events had happened in the past week that finally brought Joe to the realization that he had to make some serious changes. The first involved an afternoon golf outing. Joe had not played golf in nearly two years, but he had been invited to play by a wealthy contractor and he was eager to build a business relationship with this man. As he was unloading his bags, he asked his host where the golf carts were located and the man replied that golf carts were for sissies and that he kept in shape by walking and pulling his own cart. They had not even finished the second hole when Joe realized that the simple and seemingly easy task of casually pulling a golf cart was exhausting him. He did his best to hide his fatigue, but his host noticed his labored breathing and asked him if he were okay. Joe replied, "Of course, allergy season, gets me every year," and the host accepted the lie and they continued playing.

Joe survived the golf game but three days later he was working in his yard when his retired neighbor walked across the street and asked for his assistance in moving a piece of heavy furniture from his house to his garage. "I need about three guys to move it, but I figure you're stronger than any three guys in the neighborhood so I thought I would just ask you," said the neighbor. Joe smiled; even at his age it was still nice to be thought of in those terms. He lifted the heavy armoire easily enough, but by the time he got done carrying it less than 50 feet, he was winded and gasping for breath. Again, he dismissed the concerned neighbor by explaining that he had been fighting the flu for several days and had not been sleeping well and that he was fine and probably just needed to catch up on some sleep.

Joe reflected on those events with disgust. He had finally had enough. He

> HE STILL LOOKED FIT AND STRONG ON THE OUTSIDE, BUT INTERNALLY HE FELT TERRIBLE.

pulled out a yellow legal pad from his desk and began outlining a plan to get back into shape. He would increase his water intake and would begin packing healthful lunches; he would add more volume to his strength workouts; and most importantly of all, he would get up four mornings a week and either run or bike for several miles. Joe knew from experience that if he did not do it first thing in the morning, it would not get done. It was easy to plan to run in the evening before or after dinner, but something always seemed to get in the way. He also promised to engage his sons in pickup basketball games in the evenings and on weekends. He vowed to do this come hell or high water. He tore the sheet off the legal pad and placed it in his day planner and smiled. He knew this plan would have him back in shape in no time at all.

Joe's alarm went off at 5:00 a.m. the following morning. He quickly turned it off so as to not wake his sleeping wife and sat up in the bed. A hard, driving rain was beating against the bedroom window. Joe quickly concluded that perhaps it was best to postpone his morning training; after all, it was dangerous to run or bike in this kind of weather and it just felt so good to sleep in a bit during an early morning rain. He vowed to make up for it the next day. The following day brought rain as well. Each day Joe promised himself that the next day he would get up and run.

Two months went by and every time that Joe saw the folded paper in his day planner it angered him more. He had finally had enough, he was going to get up and exercise the following Monday no matter what. He set the alarm for 5:00 a.m. and carefully laid out his running gear for the following day. He would not be deterred from starting this program.

The alarm went off at 5:00 a.m. but Joe did not respond to the noise. He had died in his sleep at 3:17 a.m. of congestive heart failure, according to the autopsy reports.

His funeral was held three days later and people came from miles around to pay their respects. Whispers of "how could this have happened, he was in such good shape?" emanated from the small groups of people huddled in the church foyer prior to the memorial service. Joe's family was ushered to their seats, but rather than sitting down, Marie tearfully approached the open casket. She steadied herself with one hand on the railing and she reached out and lightly touched the lapel of Joe's suit. "Why, Joe, why?" she gasped as the crowd in attendance choked back tears. "Joe, why . . . why?"

> JOE KNEW FROM EXPERIENCE THAT IF HE DID NOT DO IT FIRST THING IN THE MORNING, IT WOULD NOT GET DONE.

Marie placed her other hand on Joe's shoulders and gently shook him. "Joe why . . . why did you set the alarm for five a.m.?" Joe sat up in bed, startled but relieved to be out of the nightmare he was having. He quickly turned off the alarm clock and got out of bed. "Sorry, Marie," he said, "I am going to go out for a run this morning." "In this weather?" asked Marie. "It's pouring outside, come back to bed and run tomorrow when the weather is nicer." Joe quickly dressed and kissed his wife on the forehead. "Go back to sleep darling, I won't be long." He stepped out of the house and faced the early morning wind and rain. Joe took a long breath and began running for his life. M

# Medicine Ball Throws to Increase Power and Quickness

### Col. (Ret.) Joseph H. Wolfenberger

**M**any of you probably think of pairs of wrestlers, boxers, or martial artists throwing medicine balls back and forth when the subject of training with this equipment comes up. There's nothing wrong with that concept, but in this article I want to explain two exercises which can be performed by one person and bring great physical benefits.

You'll need at least one medicine ball, available at most athletic supply stores. I have two balls, 9-lb. and 12-lb., which give more flexibility and variety, but I used only one for a long time with good results. I might add here that if you don't want to purchase a medicine ball, a round-shaped rock weighing 8 to 12 lb. (or heavier, if you prefer) will work just as well. I train with rocks also to add variety. If you do go that route, I recommend that you wear some leather work gloves.

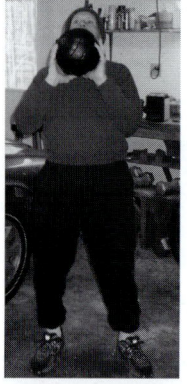

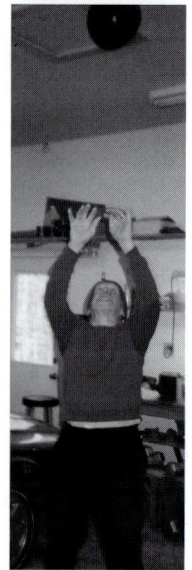

**Overhanded medicine ball throw, start and toss.**
Photos courtesy of Joseph Wolfenberger.

### Exercises

1. *Underhanded throw.* Stand with the ball between your legs, hands in the palms-up position, feet about shoulder-width apart, and knees slightly bent. Forcibly extend the legs and throw the ball directly overhead in one explosive movement. Catch the ball and repeat for 8 to 10 reps (more or less if you prefer). Continue for a second and third set. You may want to experiment with reps and sets to see what works best for you.

If I am using a rock, I will frequently just let it land on the ground, pick it up, and go for another rep. If you do the exercise in this way, you'll soon see progress because you'll be throwing the ball (or rock) higher and will feel increased power and quickness.

2. *Overhanded throw.* Stand with the ball in your hands in the upright position (as in the military press starting position), with the knees slightly bent and the feet about shoulder-width apart. Straighten your knees and arms in one explosive movement and push the ball straight overhead. Do 6 to 8 reps for the first set and repeat for 2 more sets, adding or decreasing reps for subsequent sets as needed. For variety, you can split the legs in the finish position (as in the split jerk). Experiment a little to find the sets and reps that work best for you. Again, after a few workouts you'll be pushing the ball higher, and you'll begin to notice other changes in your physical status. I might add that you'll also be sucking air if you do 10 reps or so for 3 sets of this exercise.

You'll soon see the many benefits of performing just these two exercises with a medicine ball or rock: increased overall power in the arms, shoulders, legs, and wrists; increased jerking and snatching power with a barbell or dumbbells; increased jumping ability; and improved coordination and quickness, which will enhance overall athletic performance.

Having tried many different methods to preserve or increase my performance as an athlete and weight trainer through the years, I found a technique which has significantly enhanced my capability on the above two exercises. Most readers of *MILO* have performed shoulder shrugs sometime during their training days, either with a barbell or dumbbells. I regularly perform this exercise, and quite by accident I found that by consciously and vigorously shrugging the shoulders, activating the trapezius and other muscles in the area, while tossing the medicine ball—or while doing cleans, jerks, snatches—I could exert substantially more force.

Being a karate practitioner, I have also found that the shrugging movement adds significantly to my punching and blocking technique and power. I emphasize that this shrugging action of the shoulders must be forceful and vigorous to be effective. I believe you must have practiced the shoulder shrug movement fairly recently in your training program to have the coordination required to apply the motion while performing these other exercises. This shrugging technique may sound like voodoo or be old hat to some of you out there, but if you aren't familiar with it, do give it a try.

I believe you'll find these two medicine ball exercises will make significant contributions to your training progress. **M**

> I EMPHASIZE THAT THIS SHRUGGING ACTION OF THE SHOULDERS MUST BE FORCEFUL AND VIGOROUS TO BE EFFECTIVE.

# IRON FILINGS

**Randall J. Strossen, Ph.D.** | *Publisher & Editor-in-chief*

Top German weightlifting coach Frank Mantek assessed his team's performance at the recent European Weightlifting Championships, both in itself and as a stepping stone to this year's World Weightlifting Championships and the 2012 Olympics. Mantek said, "Now the European Championships in 2010 are a history . . . with one silver and two bronze medals we have won with our Olympic champion Matthias Steiner and his training companion Almir Velagic a total of three medals in Minsk.

"In particular for Matthias Steiner this competition was a very important landmark, his first appearance after his spectacular Olympic victory of Peking 2008. If one compares [his] results of the Olympic Games (461 kg) and now in Minsk (426 kg), one could reach to the result that this appearance was relatively bad. I as his longstanding coach see this, nevertheless, a little bit different." Mantek went on to make three important points about Steiner's results at the Europeans and what they meant:

"First, we have fulfilled our [main goal] with a medal in the total. Second, it is obvious that we have currently clear deficits, in particular in the technical area in the snatch. 190 kg is not enough for a realistic fight for international titles. Third,

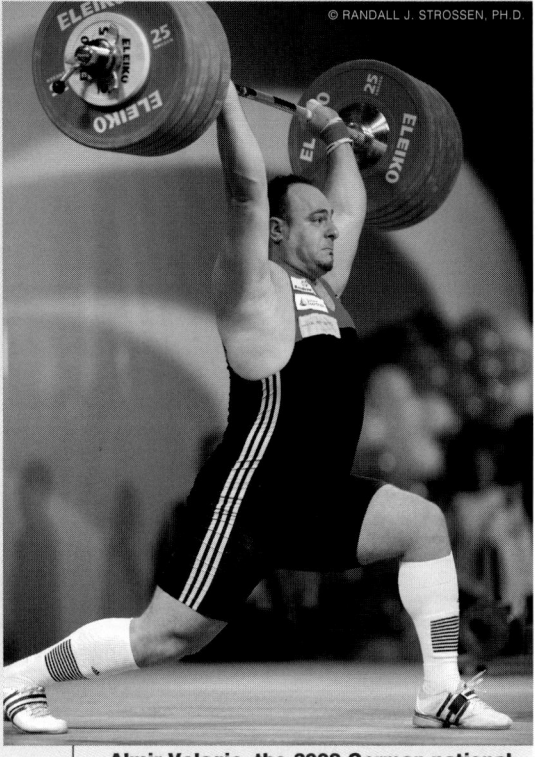

**Almir Velagic, the 2009 German national champion in the snatch, stuck this personal record 235-kg clean and jerk at the 2010 European Weightlifting Championships.**
Randall J. Strossen photo.

Matthias showed with his last attempt in the clean and jerk (251 kg) that he still is [in a position to] fight for the gold medal. It is necessary for it that we gain control of his present deficits in the snatch."

Mantek feels that Matthias is capable of doing what it takes to come out on top again: "This ability distinguishes true champions and Matthias is whole without doubt one of this species."

"In preparation for the 2010 World Championships, we have planned a lot of training camps beyond our home training center Leimen (not far from Heidelberg, the present hometown of Matthias). Besides the traditional training camps within Germany, longer training phases are also planned in Paris, Madrid and Tenerife. I am very confident that we will play a very important role at the [2010 Worlds]. Our second starter in the super heavyweight class, Almir Velagic, set a new personal best with 425 kg in Minsk. Keep to us the fingers crossed that everybody stays healthy." M

Chances are that if you are passionate enough about strength to be reading MILO, you might like to share your thoughts, questions and opinions with fellow enthusiasts—especially with the other people who read this journal. You are now able to do just that because IronMind recently launched a forum, so consider this your invitation to stop by, have a virtual beverage or two, and exchange ideas with a very special slice of the strength world.

Olympic-style weightlifting, grip, strongman, stones, Highland Games—if it has to do with strength and you want to talk about it, stop by to ask a question or state an opinion. The IronMind Forum will give you a home to pursue your passion.

Open, real names—no place for wizards of odd or serial flame throwers—this could be just your kind of place if MILO rings your bell. Navigate from the IronMind homepage by just clicking on the IronMind Forum button or go directly to www.ironmindforum.com.

If you love weightlifting, you'll want to check out the IronMind Big Lift Series on YouTube. There you can see clips of world champions like Marc Huster, Naim Suleymanoglu, Pyrros Dimas, Ivan Chakarov, and most recently, Stefan Botev, doing just what it says . . . big lifts. The latest video added is Botev's 245-kg clean and jerk from the 1995 World Weightlifting Championships. Andrei Chemerkin, Ronny Weller and Stefan Botev —they would duel for medals at the 1996 Olympics and the stage was set one year earlier at the world championships in Guangzhou, China. Stop by, take a look . . . and get inspired. M

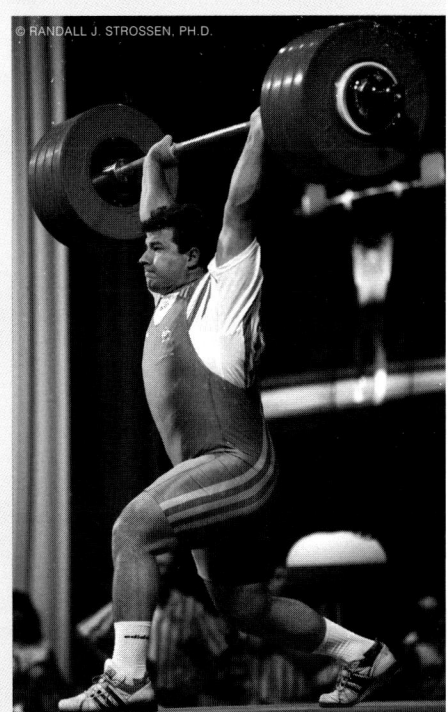

At the 1996 Olympics, Stefan Botev opened with this 240-kg clean and jerk. The run-up to the Olympics began at the 1995 World Weightlifting Championships, where Botev cleaned and jerked 245 kg on his third attempt.
Randall J. Strossen photo.

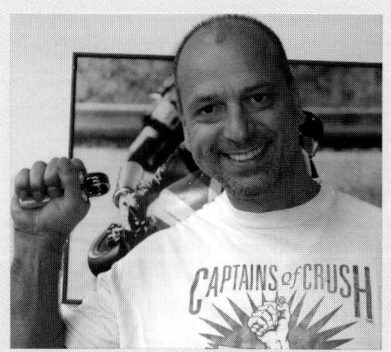

Manfred Hoeberl still has his original Captains of Crush T-shirt from the 1990s . . . when he nearly closed a No. 3 gripper on sight and would subsequently go on to get certified after audibly clicking the handles together.
Photo courtesy of Manfred Hoeberl.

**H**e had 25-inch arms and the sort of physique that would have been easy to dismiss Manfred Hoeberl as being a mere bodybuilder, but it only took a few minutes of watching him compete at the 1994 European Musclepower Championship to realize that he really was a strongman—and we would soon find out why everyone talked about Manfred Hoeberl's grip strength.

As we described it in the January 1995 (Vol. 2, No. 4) issue of MILO: ". . . we had the opportunity to let Manfred Hoeberl give one of our #3 grippers a squeeze. On first sight, with no warm-up or chalk, Manfred laid out the most serious squeeze we have ever witnessed under comparable conditions—bringing the handles down to about 1/8-inch of each other. We are used to seeing really strong guys get the handles down to about 3/4-inch, but anyone who hits the last 1/4-inch or better on his first try makes a very big impression on us" (p. 26).

Since then, Manfred has used up some of his nine lives in both car and motorcycle accidents, but his prodigious hand strength remains. Although he has not really trained in years, Manfred Hoeberl recently picked up a No. 2 Captains of Crush Gripper and closed it on sight. Want more? Manfred told Randall Strossen that he will train a little on the grippers and, if so, our money is on him to once again click a No. 3.

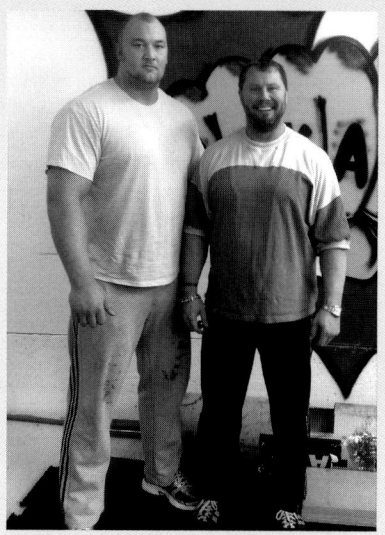

Hafþór Júlíus Björnsson (l.), standing 2.05 meters (nearly 6' 9") tall, and weighing 170 kg, nearly dwarfs four-time World's Strongest Man winner Magnus Ver Magnusson (r.).
Photo courtesy of Magnus Ver Magnusson.

"**H**ey Randall, here is a picture of my new Icelandic strongman giant!!!" four-time World's Strongest Man winner Magnus Ver Magnusson emailed to MILO publisher Randall Strossen. "I found him last year. He is 21 years old and is over 170 kg now . . . give me a call."

Magnus Ver Magnusson, president of the Federation of Icelandic Strongmen, told us that Hafþór Júlíus Björnsson used to play basketball, and the two met shortly before Magnus Ver Magnusson opened his gym, Jakabol. A knee injury ended Björnsson's basketball career, Magnusson said, but he seemed like a good prospect for strongman. In fact, Björnsson broke two Icelandic records in the stone carry last year and, along with gaining about 35 kg of bodyweight since their initial meeting, Björnsson is now deadlifting 350 kg.

"In two years he will be really good," Magnusson said of his latest find. M

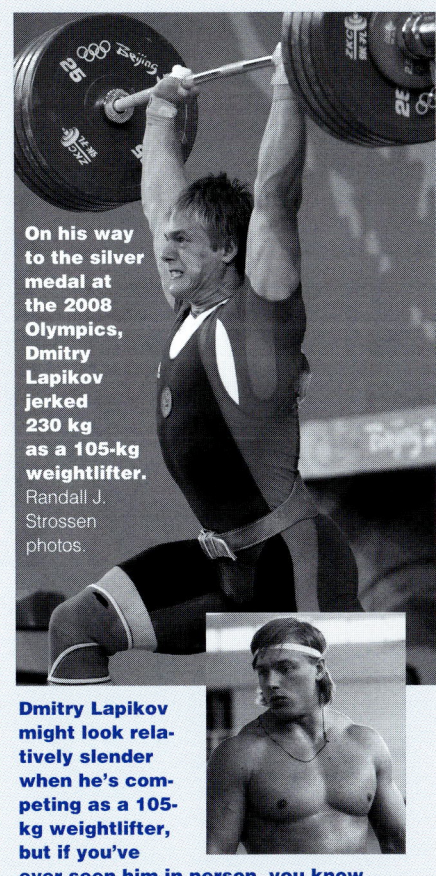

On his way to the silver medal at the 2008 Olympics, Dmitry Lapikov jerked 230 kg as a 105-kg weightlifter.
Randall J. Strossen photos.

Dmitry Lapikov might look relatively slender when he's competing as a 105-kg weightlifter, but if you've ever seen him in person, you know how muscular he is.

With great sadness, MILO received word in April from his family that Lee Gesbeck passed away. Lee was part of MILO for many years and was the person who early on championed our coverage of all-round lifting, becoming our principal reporter on all-round records. Lee also had a special interest in World's Strongest Man and would often be one of the first people to ask for details about the forthcoming World's Strongest Man contest. He consistently wrote to thank us for whatever coverage we included as the contest was taking place.

Lee had iron in his veins and we'll miss his phone calls and emails. May he rest in peace. M

As a 105-kg weightlifter, Russia's Dmitry Lapikov is hardly a slouch: he regularly snatches at least 190 kg, and at the 2008 Olympics, he cleaned and jerked 230 kg. For all his success, though, Lapikov is looking for bigger things, and the cornerstone of his plans is moving up to the +105-kg category.

Lapikov told MILO that he is currently weighing about 113 kg and that he would like to compete at about 130 kg bodyweight. This reporter expressed the opinion that the increase in bodyweight might help his jerks, and

Lapikov agreed. While impressively muscular and solid in person, Lapikov looks almost slender on the competition platform. Since he's already proven himself to have world-class pulling power at 105-kg bodyweight, if more mass and a bigger core help his jerks, he might be a very hard man for anyone to beat. M

**D**r. Dominik Doerr, a member of the European Weightlifting Federation Medical Committee, has shared with MILO data on injuries at the European and World Weightlifting Championships, as well as at the Olympic Games—and for anyone who thinks weightlifting is a dangerous sport, the data prove otherwise.

Once upon a time, there was a feeling was that lifting weights would make you slow and inflexible, and that it would even stunt your growth. Such claims might sound silly today, since virtually all top athletes include resistance training in their workouts, but what of injuries? Especially in the Olympic sport of weightlifting where huge weights are snatched or cleaned and jerked in the blink of an eye, isn't this just an open invitation to getting hurt?

Such is not the case, and the ongoing data presented by Dominic Doerr, M.D. clearly contradict the myth that the sport of weightlifting is dangerous. And to really put a sharp point on this analysis and its conclusions, the data analyzed by Dr. Doerr were drawn from the sport's most competitive level: the Senior European Weightlifting Championships, the Senior World Weightlifting Championships, and the Olympic Games.

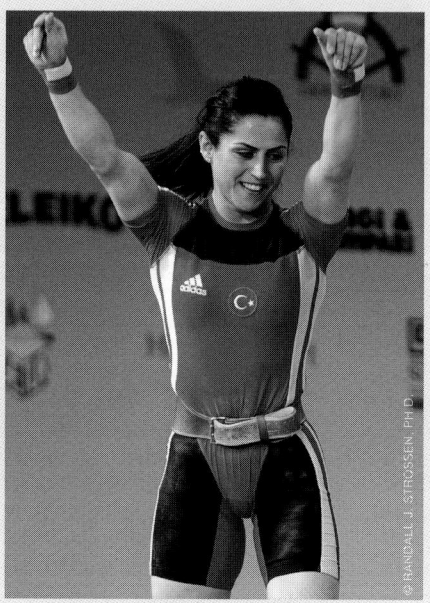

Turkish weightlifting star Sibel Simsek quietly celebrates a good lift at the 2008 European Weightlifting Championships (Lignano-Sabbiadoro, Italy). Lifting in the women's 63-kg category, Simsek snatched 105 kg, and cleaned and jerked 121 kg.
Randall J. Strossen photo.

"If you look to the data, some things are already obvious," Dr. Doerr remarked as he summarized the principal conclusions about who gets injured and when:

• men have more injuries than women
• lighter bodyweight categories seem to be more "dangerous"
• the elbow is the most affected body part
• second and third attempts have more injuries (which is simply logic), but there seems to be a cue that in the snatch, it is the second attempt, but in the clean and jerk, the third one

Strike another myth about weightlifting, because the truth is that it has a "low risk of injury," Dr. Doerr said. M

Although he's long since been retired from strongman competition, 2001 World's Strongest Man winner Svend "Viking" Karlsen rocked the strength world when he casually talked about working up to a 400-kg deadlift this summer. Recently Viking told MILO that he has shelved the heavy deadlifts for the moment, but what's this: arms that are getting close to 23 inches? Viking said that he is weighing 139 or 140 kg at the moment and is aiming to weigh about 130 kg this summer.

"I am getting into good shape, training purely like a bodybuilder. If I can't be strong, I'm at least going to look like I am strong," he quipped. On the heavy deadlifts, Karlsen said that he had to back off because of his joints and has kept them light for months now, although he is squatting 500 lb. for eight reps, rock bottom and squeezing the reps out like a bodybuilder. With no end in sight for him, Viking said, "I have been training now for 30 years and it is like my religion, my church." M

World's Strongest Man and *Dancing With the Stars* winner Magnus Samuelsson is a straightforward, modest man, so when he says, "100 kg for curls doesn't feel like a lot to me," it's simple fact, not braggadocio.

Samuelsson, who's also been dubbed the owner of The World's Strongest Arms, said that after a hectic schedule left him with little time or energy to train, he's been getting back in the gym the last few months and progress has been good.

Toward the end of his competitive career as a strongman, back problems plagued the popular Swedish powerhouse: "First, it bothered me on deadlifts and squats, but then it got worse. If I was walking around and dropped something, I had to stop and think about bending down to pick it up," Samuelsson explained.

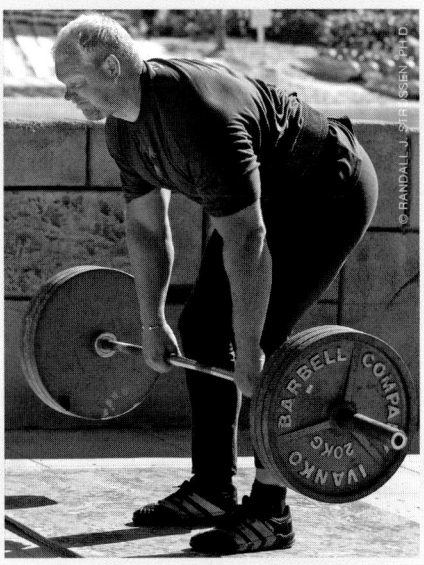

**Magnus Samuelsson warms up with some deadlifts at the 2004 World's Strongest Man contest.**
Randall J. Strossen photo.

Three and half months ago, Samuelsson said he couldn't deadlift 200 kg, but now he can do a few reps with 300 kg "quite easily," and as part of his training, he deadlifts while standing on three 25-kg plates to increase the range of motion. Samuelsson said that he is also doing front squats again as part of his training.

Weighing 146 kg, Samuelsson has arms bigger and stronger than most men's legs, and Samuelsson said that his basic biceps routine has been the same for 20 years, built around barbell curls: 60 kg x 15 reps, 80 kg x 15 reps, 100 kg x 15 reps, and if he feels good, back to 60 kg x 15 reps.

"This involves some grip training," Samuelsson said, who has always used a straight bar for curls so that he can let the bar roll as far down toward his fingertips as possible before bringing it back into his hand, curling his wrists, and then continuing the movement.

"Can you still just pick up a No. 3 Captains of Crush Gripper and close it?" MILO asked.

"I like to think it's like riding a bike—I've never forgotten," he said. M

## NAHA Season Kick-off
by Thom Van Vleck

Shreveport, Louisiana

The 2010 North American Highlander Association's (NAHA) season is off to a big start: so far this year there are 10 meets scheduled before the end of July. Last year's season ended with the Scarecrow Festival Highlander October 3 and the Lift for Hope Highlander on October 17, which meant there were 9 contests in NAHA's inaugural year, so 2010 is heating up for NAHA. The meets that are entering their second year are having increased participation, and the enthusiasm continues to grow as we gear up for the Nationals in Omaha, Nebraska on July 31. This meet will have even larger cash prizes than last year and is looking to be a well-sponsored meet.

The season kicked-off with a contest on March 6 in Shreveport, Louisiana, where there is a lot of enthusiasm for the Highlander concept, a combination of Highland Games and strongman events. The next meet was the Missouri State Highlander held on March 27 in Kirksville. This meet was hosted by the Jackson Weightlifting Club and one of the events was the anvil clean and press; of course, the anvil was the legendary Grandpa Jackson's Anvil.

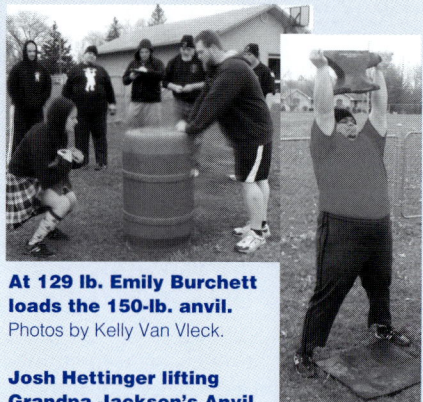

At 129 lb. Emily Burchett loads the 150-lb. anvil.
Photos by Kelly Van Vleck.

Josh Hettinger lifting Grandpa Jackson's Anvil at the Missouri State Highlander.

April 10 brought the Brute Strength Gym Highlander in Norfolk, Virginia. Sporting sponsorship from IronMind, VPX, and Optimum Nutrition, with bagpipes playing and Barry Von Perkins as the emcee, this contest had a big-time feel. The following week brought the Global Gilbert Festival Highlander in Arizona on April 17; it was a hot and sunny day with plenty of sunburns for everyone. May 2 brought the Western New York Highlander, which featured a very large middleweight class.

The contests thus far have had close battles, big throws, tiebreakers and tight races and more excitement is expected. The future of NAHA is looking very bright. M

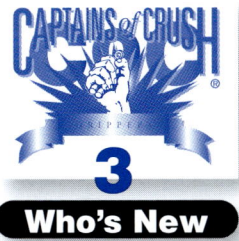

## Who's New

Two gripsters have conquered the No. 3 Captains of Crush Gripper—one of them for the second time!—and have been added to the certified list:

Craig Call
Paul Knight

For a complete list of those certified on the No. 3, No. 3.5, and No. 4 Captains of Crush Grippers, or for the Rules for Closing and Certification, please visit the IronMind website at **www.ironmind.com**.

Craig Call, of Ashland, Ohio, is 20 years old, and the 6' 2" 250-lb. Ashland University hammer thrower and shot putter is coached by no less than 4-time Olympian Jud Logan.

"My grip training has had a direct positive influence on my throwing and lifting numbers," Craig said. He trains grip "three times a week. A typical gripper workout consists of progressively harder gripper closes, a couple of credit card sets with the No. 3, and then with the No. 3.5, which I have closed several times. I would like to thank my teammates, family, girlfriend Jayne, and coaches for all of their positive support and enthusiasm. A special thank you goes to judge Howard Liviskie for donating his free time to make my certification attempt a success."

Of Craig, Howard said, "I was very impressed by Craig's hand strength, but I was more impressed by his energy and his very apparent love for strength training and grip strength."

Welcome to the club, Craig! M

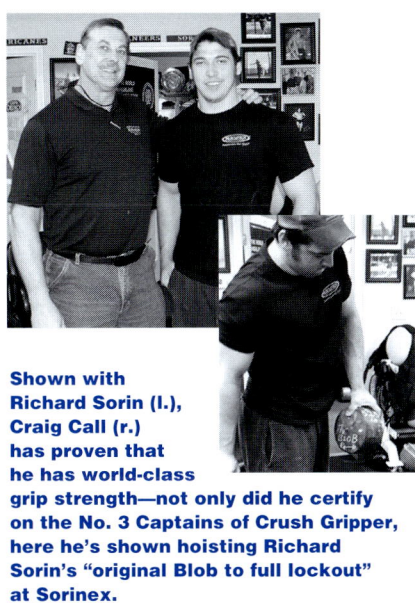

**Shown with Richard Sorin (l.), Craig Call (r.) has proven that he has world-class grip strength**—not only did he certify on the No. 3 Captains of Crush Gripper, here he's shown hoisting Richard Sorin's "original Blob to full lockout" at Sorinex.
Photos courtesy of Craig Call.

Thirty-two-year-old Paul Knight of Fort Worth, Texas, who stands 6' tall and weighs 225 lb., told us:

"I certified on the No. 3 in 2003 and recently decided to re-certify under the rule change," referring to the change in 2004 that defined a legal starting position to be at least the width of a credit/ATM card. "I saw that Richard Sorin had re-certified so I thought I [would] do the same as it is a more difficult close from the credit card width versus the old 1" rule. In addition, I could get a little

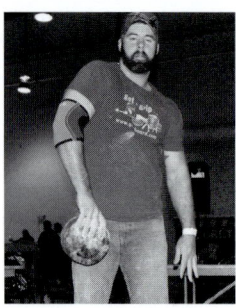

Paul Knight, shown here lifting the Blob, has re-certified on the No. 3 Captains of Crush Gripper.
Photo courtesy of Joe Musselwhite.

extra practice for when I attempt the No. 3.5."

Paul tries to "train grip 2 times per week if I'm injury free . . . pinch grip, support grip, and grippers. Steel bending is another grip-related form of exercise I like to work on and I have been certified on the Red Nail."

Congratulations to Paul Knight, whose name has been added (again) to the official No. 3 Captains of Crush certification list, and a special thanks to Danny Peters for helpfully serving as Paul's official referee. M

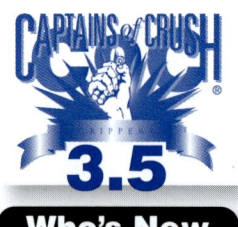

### Who's New

Two men already certified on the No. 3 Captains of Crush Gripper upped the ante, crushing the formidable No. 3.5 CoC:

Jonathan Vogt
Paul Knight

For a complete list of those certified on the No. 3, No. 3.5, and No. 4 Captains of Crush Grippers, or for the Rules for Closing and Certification, please visit the IronMind website at www.ironmind.com.

**J**onathan Vogt first hit MILO's radar when he certified on the No. 3 Captains of Crush Gripper as a mere 19-year-old. We couldn't help but be interested in the story of this young man who had started mowing lawns to earn money and had built up a lawn care business while he attended classes at Purdue University, and who attributed a lot of grip strength to the work he did behind his Scag mower.

That was just a warm-up because Jonathan Vogt has also certified on the No. 3.5 Captains of Crush Gripper, the youngest person to date to reach this huge milestone in the grip strength world.

"I am 20 years old [and] am 6' 1", 260 lb. at this time. I still do my mowing and landscaping which greatly involves my hands," Jonathan said. "I have close to 1,000 hours of mowing time on my one Scag, which builds my hands. I keep my grippers in my truck and in my pockets at all times. I close them as much as I can almost every day. I think this is the secret to building

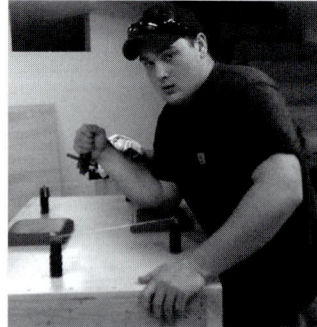

Jonathan Vogt is on a roll. He ran through the No. 3 Captains of Crush Gripper and now the No. 3.5, so you know what's coming next.
Photo courtesy of Jonathan Vogt.

hand strength: using your hands everyday in some form of a challenge, no matter what it is. I am very close to closing the No. 4, and I would also like to certify on the Red Nail. I enjoy seeing that every Captains of Crush Gripper is almost identical . . ."

Congratulations, Jonathan, your name has been added to the official certification list for the No. 3.5 Captains of Crush Gripper. MILO would also like to say a special thanks to John Hight, retired USAF, for graciously serving as Jonathan Vogt's official referee. M

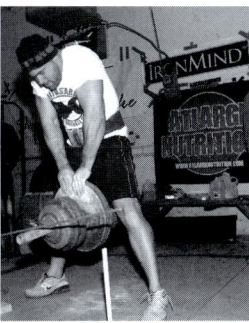

If you think you just read about Paul Knight, you're right, because Paul has re-certified on the No. 3 CoC in this issue as well as certifying for the first time on the No. 3.5. For more on Paul, please see his profile on pp. 77–78.

Congratulations, Paul; you'll find your name on the No. 3.5 Captains of Crush certified list. Many thanks to Eric Milfeld, himself certified on both the No. 3 and the Red Nail, who agreed on short notice to serve as Paul's referee as Paul told us, "I am peaking in my hand strength at the moment." M

# CALENDAR

Check out the Latest News at **www.ironmind.com**, the Strength World's News Source.

**2010 NA Strongman, Inc.**
Sept 4   Mass. State Championships, Everett, MA
Oct 30   The Training Box Strongman Contest, Fort Meyers, FL
Nov 12   NAS National Championships North America's Strongest Man, Reno, NV

For upcoming contest and information, visit www.nastrongman-inc.com or contact Willie and Dione Wessels, 314-770-9279, email: dione@americanstrongman.com.

**2010 United States Armwrestling Association, Inc.**
Oct 2   2010 Missouri State AW Championships, O'Fallon, MO
Nov 13   5th Annual Kentucky Muscle AW Challenge, Louisville, KY
Dec 4–11   WAF World AW Championships, Mesquite, NV

For more information, contact the USAA, 246 Custer Avenue, Billings, MT 59101; 406-248-4508 or 406-245-1560; www.usarmwrestling.com.

**2010 United States All-Round W/L Assn.**
For upcoming events and information, contact Bill Clark, 3906 Grace Ellen Drive, Columbia, MO 652021796. USAWA is a drug-free organization.

**2010 Powerlifting**
For scheduled events, check *Powerlifting USA* magazine. For subscription information, call 800-448-7693 or 805-482-2378.

**2010 USA Weightlifting/IWF**
Sep 18–30   World WL Championships, Antalya, Turkey
Oct 3–14   Commonwealth Games, Delhi, India
Nov 12–27   Asian Games, Guangzhou, China
Dec 10–12   American Open, Cincinnati, OH

For more information on USA Weightlifting contests, please contact 719-866-4508 or go to www.usaweightlifting.org. For information about international competitions, please visit www.iwf.net.

**2010 Highland Games**
For schedules of competitions, please see the following websites:
- www.nasgaweb.com
- www.asgf.org
- www.saaa-net.org
- www.highlandnet.com

# How to Live a Lot in
# One Day

**Myles Wetzel**

**M**any people wonder why anyone would compete in a Highland Games: you do seven events in one day and it is very demanding. At the end of the day you even have trouble sleeping sometimes, you are so sore and tired. I suppose the challenge of competing and completing such a day is part of the reason. The great Teddy Roosevelt addressed this so clearly in his speech "Citizenship in a Republic" at the Sorbonne, Paris, 23 April 1910:

"It is not the critic who counts: not the man who points out how the strong man stumbles or where the doer of deeds could have done better. The credit belongs to the man who is actually in the arena, whose face is marred by dust and sweat and blood, who strives valiantly, who errs and comes up short again and again, because there is no effort without error or shortcoming, but who knows the great enthusiasms, the great devotions, who spends himself for a worthy cause; who at the best knows in the end the triumph of high achievement, and who at the worst if he fails, at least he fails while daring greatly, so that his place shall never be with those cold and timid souls who knew neither victory nor defeat."

> BY WEDNESDAY YOU'RE ALREADY STARTING TO GET THE BUZZ JUST THINKING ABOUT THE CONTEST.

When you compete in a Highland Games, most of the time it is on a Saturday. As the week leading up to the Games progresses, so does your excitement and anxiety—you're going to be on the field laying it all on the line for everyone to see. By Wednesday you're already starting to get the buzz just thinking about the contest. Thursday you're getting all your stuff ready. Friday is travel day and you get on the road and arrive in the city of the Games. That evening you have a pre-game dinner with some friends who are there to compete with you. The Highland Games community is small and everyone knows each other, and the camaraderie is part of the beauty of this sport. You plan your season to see certain people and spend the day battling with them on the field. Friday night's sleep does not come easy—you're really jacked up thinking what the next day will bring.

If he is not there, my friend Craig Smith calls me early the morning of the Games and tells me, "It is a beautiful day to throw." And he is always right. If we are rooming together at a Games, he will be up at the crack of dawn, throwing the door to the room open and proclaiming it to the world. It is a wonderful way to start any day.

You get up, bustling with excitement about the day in front of you, get dressed in your game gear, and then go get a pre-game meal of some good solid food to last you through the morning portion of the day's events. We are talking about big men with a lot of big throwing to do, so you have to eat pretty big. There are no weight classes at the Games, just big dudes throwing heavy things a long way . . . and that takes a lot of energy.

You arrive at the field and can't wait to jump out of the truck and hit the grass, get in the athletes' tent, and get ready. We put on our shoes and kilt for the first event and start to warm up and get moving. We meet the judges and make sure we are signed up and ready to start.

The Games start early and follow a traditional order. Once you step over the rope onto the field of honor, there is no hiding and the results are immediate. You get three attempts at an event. You go up and take your attempt, and the referees measure and announce it. Everyone completes the three attempts and the event is over. You complete one event and move on to the next. There is no waiting around or contemplating your next move—you give it all you have and then move on. The day flies by.

It is hard to be good in seven events, so your day has ups and downs, but no matter what, you are on the field and giving it your all. In the blink of an eye you complete the fourth event, the hammer, and it is time for lunch. The athletes are provided a lunch with plenty of drinks all day to keep them hydrated. You have just completed the hammer so there is tacky all over your hands. You never seem to get tacky off when you want to—it is always on the cell phone, the steering wheel, and your clothing. The stuff sticks, but hey, is that not what you use it for? Ah, we love the smell of tacky. It is a pine tar blend that is widely celebrated. It helps keep you attached to things you're throwing: they are so heavy that the force is more than the grips of even the strongest men can handle.

> YOU NEVER SEEM TO GET TACKY OFF WHEN YOU WANT TO—IT IS ALWAYS ON THE CELL PHONE, THE STEERING WHEEL, AND YOUR CLOTHING.

After a short lunch break comes the favorite event of most spectators, the caber. It is the most well-known of the events and the crowds seem to enjoy it the most. Each Games has a different caber that was cut down and prepared for the Games that year. It is really a tree. You hold it upright with the small end in your hand and run and throw it and hopefully it turns over when it hits the ground. It is an event of accuracy, not distance or height. You are trying to turn it straight away from you and the results are measured like the face of a clock. A 12:00 landing position is perfection. If the caber lands just a little to the right of straight ahead of you, that is 1:00. A little to the left and it is 11:00. Again, you have three tries at this toss.

Now, caber theory is different around the country. In some areas they want to see a lot of guys turning the caber, with the results deciding who is the best. In other areas they want to have a stick so big only one or two men can turn it. So depending on the Games, you can have a lighter shootout caber, or a giant of a pole that pulls your arms out of their sockets.

After the caber is completed, there are two height events and then the day is complete. Points are tallied to determine who the athlete of the day is, and medals and swords are handed out. The winner of a Highland Games gets a weapon of death—nothing is coveted more than the big sword for the athlete of the day. You keep that in a place of honor in your home, or even one of them in the truck, just to get the good feeling from it whenever you like. One look at the sword and a flood of memories from that day come into your mind and you relish and rehash the day. It is a glorious feeling like no other. It is a shame that few men get this wonderful feeling in life—if you could bottle that feeling and sell it, people might give their souls for it.

After the medals and swords are handed out, all the athletes go back to the hotels. Many meet up for a huge post-game celebratory meal and start to relive the day and decompress after the excitement. Everyone at the table feels like a king. You see, there are no losers in a Highland Games event. All the men won that day—they met the challenge and did the deed. They laid it all out on the field of honor for everyone to see and gave it their all and completed the day. They feel so alive and victorious. There is no feeling in the world like that after completing a Highland Games event—you feel as if you lived five days in one. So much happened, there was so much emotion and feeling: the afterglow of a Games day is so grand.

The following day start the post-game thoughts. You sit in silence and play each event, throw, and result over and over in your mind. Each thing said and each laugh from the day is repeated in your mind like a computer as you relive the day, remembering the fabulous time you had. No matter how hard your day was, how tough the competition, "We also glory in tribulations, knowing that tribulations produce perseverance" (Romans 5:3–5). I can only assume that is one of the reasons you will find a person who competes in the Highland Games to be one of the toughest, most enduring friends you can have on this earth.

If you ever have an interest, take the chance. Try the Games—you will live more in one day than you have ever before.

> EVERYONE AT THE TABLE FEELS LIKE A KING. YOU SEE, THERE ARE NO LOSERS IN A HIGHLAND GAMES EVENT.

# Those Awesome Antioxidants

## Bill Starr

Author of *The Strongest Shall Survive: Strength Training for Football* and *Defying Gravity*

Good health is the prerequisite for obtaining greater strength and overall fitness. This truism is, however, constantly overlooked as aspiring strength athletes seek methods to help them obtain their goals. They spend a great deal of time and money chasing after the elusive magic elixir that will move them to higher and higher levels of strength, while they ignore the information available that can help them to stay healthy.

There are many reasons why progress comes to a halt. Injuries and illnesses top the list. Warming up properly and using correct form can eliminate the vast majority of injuries that plague strength athletes, and understanding the usefulness of a group of vitamins known as antioxidants can greatly reduce the odds of coming down with one of the numerous maladies that lurk out there today.

Think about all of the possible contagions we hear about today: influenza, bird flu, swine flu, Lyme disease, SARS, West Nile virus, mono, and strep, a wide assortment of allergies, and a couple of deadly diseases making a comeback, smallpox and tuberculosis. Plus another dozen seem to pop up overnight. And let's not forget the common cold, although this seems to be a vanishing illness. No one has a cold anymore, even if they're sneezing and coughing, and their noses are running like a fountain. Now they have allergies. I can't tell you how many times I've talked to someone on the phone and noticed how hoarse they were and said, "You need to do something about that cold," and they always reply, "It's not a cold. It's just allergies." Fine, but you're still sick. Do something for it.

> NO ONE HAS A COLD ANYMORE, EVEN IF THEY'RE SNEEZING AND COUGHING, AND THEIR NOSES ARE RUNNING LIKE A FOUNTAIN.

In fact, allergies of all sorts are on the rise, and they can be troublesome to anyone wanting to improve his physical well-being. There's seasonal pollen, smog, exhaust fumes, secondhand smoke, additives in the food we eat, and impurities in the water we drink. In addition, those who train hard and heavy carry an extra burden because they place a much greater demand on their immune systems than do a more sedentary lot.

I am well aware that even those who are diligent in taking the correct supplements and do everything in their power not to expose themselves to the multiple negatives in daily life will sometimes have the odds stacked against them and become sick. It could be due to a long period of rest deprivation, or a time of extreme mental or physical stress, or just a quirk of happenstance, like having your car break down during a pouring rain and having to walk a long distance for assistance. As Forrest Gump so aptly pointed out to all of us, s*** happens. The thing to understand is how to respond if and when it does happen.

I do my utmost not to get caught in situations that put my health in jeopardy. I eat well, exercise regularly, get ample rest (except when the Olympics or NCAAs are on very late), and take an abundance of supplements. When I was coaching at Johns Hopkins, I always greeted my favorite athletes with a handshake, and that amounted to forty or fifty athletes a day at least. I knew that it raised my risk of picking up a bug, but I washed my hands frequently and loaded up on supplements as a safeguard. For the most part that worked nicely, but every so often, while an athlete would be shaking my hand, he or she would say, "Coach, the team doctor told me not to train for a while. I have mono." Or the flu. Or strep throat. Great, why didn't they mention this before shaking my hand?

I would rush to the bathroom and give my hands a hasty scrubbing, but a couple of times a year I would come down with a cold.

No worries. As soon as I got home I would gulp down double and sometimes triple the normal dosages of antioxidants, and by morning I would be okay again. I found that the sooner I took a positive action against the invaders, the faster the illness would be cured.

> AN ANTIOXIDANT DELAYS THE PROCESS THAT TURNS CELLS RANCID.

The antioxidants, vitamins A, C, D, and E, help protect cells from the potentially damaging effects of oxygen. I've always thought it ironic that we need that precious element in order to survive, yet oxygen can also destroy our cells. An antioxidant delays the process that turns cells rancid. Our bodies need a certain amount of unsaturated fatty acids and when too much oxygen is present, this fat gets destroyed. Just as metal can rust and become useless, so can the fats inside the cells turn rancid and render those cells useless. Antioxidants also prevent oxygen from combining with other substances to form deadly hydrogen peroxide, which hastens the death of cells.

The antioxidants could also be called anti-free radicals because they take care of those as well. Free radicals are the byproducts of molecules of fat reacting with oxygen in your body—it's a natural process going on all the time. Free radicals are formed when you're exposed to any type of toxic element in the air, water, or food: first- and second-hand cigarette smoke; smog; the junk found in water, such as lead, cadmium, copper, and traces of industrial chemicals; and all the additives in food

> THAT'S THE PART MOST PEOPLE MISS. THEY HAVE THE VITAMINS, BUT FAIL TO TAKE THEM THROUGHOUT THE DAY ON A REGULAR BASIS.

(nitrates, nitrites, and the residues of pesticides and/or herbicides). Various drugs, both over-the-counter and prescription, create free radicals—even seemingly harmless aspirin. Overexposure to the sun and chronic overtraining also produce free radicals.

Sounds bleak doesn't it? It isn't. The good news is that there is something everyone can do to help himself or herself counteract all these negatives and stay in good health. It's simply a matter of purchasing some vitamins and taking them consistently. That's the part most people miss. They have the vitamins, but fail to take them throughout the day on a regular basis. It needs to be understood that when the body is under stress, the antioxidants get used up rapidly and if they're not replaced right away, that's when the body is most susceptible to illness.

I've started a few of my older friends on a supplement program, primarily because every time I saw or talked to them, they had some kind of illness. But none of them stuck with the program: they would take the vitamins for a while and then stop. When I asked them why, they responded with, "I hate taking pills," and "It's too much trouble to take them all day and night."

The result? They're now taking lots of pills, for high blood pressure, high cholesterol, depression, and so forth, and they're still sick most of the time. This, to me, is nuts. How hard is it to systematically take some supplements right after you eat and a few more times throughout the day? It's no more difficult than brushing your teeth after eating. If you can convince yourself that the supplements are indeed essential to your health and make taking them regularly a habit, it will stay with you all your life. Remember, your level of training is determined largely by your state of health so if you care about making progress, you'll pay closer attention to taking your supplements religiously.

While vitamins A, C, D, and E are usually regarded as the antioxidants, there are a couple of minerals, selenium and magnesium, that also have these properties. I will not go into the minerals in this article but will save them for another piece since I believe they deserve more attention than just a few paragraphs.

> MOST PEOPLE SIMPLY WILL NOT TAKE A MEGA DOSAGE OF VITAMIN C.

### Vitamin C

Of the antioxidants, the one that is currently receiving the most attention by far is vitamin D. I'll get to that vitamin, but want to begin with the one that I hold in the highest regard, vitamin C. It's called nature's antibiotic—and for good reason. It stops most illnesses in their tracks if the dosage is adequate. And there's the rub. Most people simply will not take a mega dosage of vitamin C. They fear that there will be some sort of terrible consequence if they do and I'm not sure why that is. The great thing about C is that it's water soluble. That means if you should take more than your body can handle, the excess is passed out through your waste.

Nobel laureate Linus Pauling, in his book *Vitamin C and the Common Cold*, brought the many benefits of the vitamin to the full attention of the masses in the early seventies. I attended one of his lectures in San Francisco and had the opportunity to chat with him afterward. I wanted to know how much he took each day and in what form. I expected him to tell me he took an exotic type of the vitamin but I was wrong. He said he used the powdered form of ascorbic acid and took no fewer than 5 grams a day. And he would double that amount should he feel the need. I've used that as my guideline ever since, although I seldom use the powdered version because the tablets are much more convenient. However, I always keep some powdered C in the refrigerator in case of emergencies. I can knock out an impending cold in a matter of hours by overdosing with it in a glass of fruit juice.

The king of mega doses of vitamin C is Dr. Robert Cathcart, an orthopedic surgeon formerly affiliated with Stanford University. He advocates large dosages of C to combat all kinds of illnesses. He once stated, "It's not that it sometimes works. It always works if the dosage is high enough." His guidelines for daily C intake are 4 to 10 grams for a healthy person, 30 to 60 grams for a minor illness, such as a common cold, and up to 100 grams for viral flu and viral pneumonia, and up to 200 grams for mononucleosis. Now that's an overdose, and few have the guts to go to that extent.

> "YOU WANT TO FLOOD YOUR CELLS WITH C AND IT WILL DESTROY THE TOXINS CAUSING YOUR FLU."

One worry is that excessive intake of vitamin C can lead to the formation of kidney stones. This has been refuted in recent research as has the rumor that excessive amounts of C in the system would produce a sort of "rebound scurvy" if a person had been taking large amounts and then stopped taking the vitamin altogether. This simply does not happen.

I used Dr. Cathcart's notion to good effect a few years ago. My training partner, Rich, had taken me to and picked me up from the airport when I went to California one winter. In return, I promised to take him and his pregnant wife out to dinner. When I called to set up a date, she answered and sounded very ill. She explained that she had some sort of flu and had been taking medication for a week with no results and was going back to the doctor the next day for another exam. She was due in just over a month and I told her it was not a good idea to be taking prescription drugs when she was that far along in her pregnancy. She asked me what she should do.

I told her to have Rich go buy some vitamin C and to take 5 grams right away and a gram every hour until she went to bed. "You want to flood your cells with C and it will destroy the toxins causing your flu. You'll know when you've taken enough when you get some lower intestinal discomfort . . . in other words, diarrhea." She groaned and I went on, "I know, diarrhea isn't pleasant, but it won't last long and it's a lot better than being sick when you're close to giving birth." She said she'd do it because she was really sick of being sick.

When I got home the next night, I called to see how she was doing. Her voice told me she was better and she was. She said she did suffer a bit of diarrhea, but by mid-morning all the flu symptoms were gone and she felt great. She cancelled the doctor's appointment and was both surprised and delighted a vitamin could do something that several potent and very expensive prescription drugs could not. I told her to keep taking 5 grams a day to ensure she would not get sick again. Then we set a date for that dinner I owed Rich.

Besides strengthening the immune system, vitamin C does a number of other things that greatly benefit anyone seeking a higher level of fitness. One of the most important functions of vitamin C is to help the body form collagen, a strong, cement-like material responsible for holding together the body's cells, including those that form muscles, tendons, ligaments, and cartilage. Collagen is also essential for maintaining solid blood vessels, strong bones, and healthy teeth.

Vitamin C works closely with calcium to build this connective tissue. Having healthy connective tissue is vital to anyone trying to increase strength or add muscular bodyweight. The walls of the various cells of the body are extremely thin, and one of the primary jobs of this connective tissue is to protect the cells from outside invaders. An adequate supply of C must be available in order to maintain this strong barrier.

Vitamin C is required for the metabolism of protein—and everyone knows how critical protein absorption is for gaining strength and size. Vitamin C is a potent enhancer of iron absorption, which in turn boosts energy levels. The B vitamins are a primary source of energy and vitamin C has to be present for the Bs to convert foods into action. Research has shown that taking at least 500 milligrams of C prior to a workout can help prevent muscle soreness. Most experts agree that an increase in free radicals that are released during strenuous exercise is the reason for sore muscles. Faster recovery translates into more progress.

Vitamin C replaces some of the hormones that are depleted during exercise, such as cortisol and epinephrine. In order for the adrenal glands to rebuild these essential hormones, there must be an adequate supply of vitamin C in the system. Keep in mind, any sort of stress—physical, mental or emotional—can destroy these hormones as well.

### Vitamin E

While there's more to say about C, I want to move on to another vitamin that I consider critical to anyone seeking to maintain good health and improve his strength, vitamin E. Like C, it's a powerful antioxidant and in addition, it is also an oxygen conservator. The latter property means that the body can utilize more oxygen during exercise. Vitamin E, in this same regard, serves as a vasodilator. Simply put, when there is a plentiful supply of E available in the system, all the various parts of the circulatory system are expanded, from the smallest arterioles and capillaries to the larger veins and

> RESEARCH HAS SHOWN THAT TAKING AT LEAST 500 MILLIGRAMS OF C PRIOR TO A WORKOUT CAN HELP PREVENT MUSCLE SORENESS.

arteries throughout the body. The benefits to the athlete should be obvious, for when the circulatory system allows blood to flow more easily through the exercising body, the workouts will go much easier.

This is why athletes are able to participate in any type of aerobic activity much longer and with more intensity after including vitamin E in their nutritional programs. While it has special merit to those who run, swim, and bike long distances, as well as to aerobic dancers and spinners, it is also beneficial to those who train with weights. Whenever a strength athlete is able to put as much energy into those final exercises in his routine as he did the first few, he is going to quickly move ahead of his competition.

One of the very best things that E does for overall health is to assist the liver in detoxifying harmful substances that we encounter every day—all those nasty toxics I identified earlier. Vitamin E is often called the sex vitamin. This came about when writers started filling the pages of the popular press with pieces about boosting virility by taking the vitamin. In truth, additional vitamin E does not increase the desire for more sexual activity nor does it improve sexual prowess. What it does do is help stimulate the production of sperm in males and help prevent miscarriages in females. Yet, by enhancing the endurance factor, it most likely will have a positive influence on the sex act. Hey, it can't hurt.

A few things need to be understood about this vitamin so you can select the best product on the shelf. Vitamin E is composed of seven forms of tocopherals, each having a letter from the Greek alphabet: alpha, beta, gamma, delta, epsilon, zeta, and eta. For some time, scientists stated that the only biologically active form of the vitamin was alpha tocopheral, but subsequent research has revealed that it's more beneficial to take all of the tocopherals together. This facilitates assimilation much better, and because this is the way they are found in nature, they should be taken in this manner. Experts do conclude, however, that alpha is the most potent of all the tocopherals.

> THE MINIMUM DAILY REQUIREMENT FOR VITAMIN E IS SO LOW IT'S LUDICROUS.

Even more important is determining whether the vitamin E comes from natural or synthetic sources. It makes a huge difference. Synthetic E is of little value, having but one-fifth of the potency of the natural form. The prefix before the listing of the various tocopherals found in the product designates whether it's natural or synthetic. The prefix dl- signifies that it's from synthetic sources and d- tells you that it's derived from natural sources. If the product is cheap, more than likely it's synthetic, so check the label closely. That bargain may not be a bargain after all.

The minimum daily requirement for vitamin E is so low it's ludicrous. Most of these standards were set before World War II and do not take into account body size or activity level. For example, a 150-lb. pound man who never exercises is allotted the same requirement as the 200-lb. pound man who trains hard and does aerobics for a total of two hours every day. I recommend a minimum of 1,200 IU of natural vitamin E per day, and 1,600 to 2,000 if the need is there—after a long illness or surgery or when someone is under a great deal of stress, for example. Take your supplement with a dairy product to aid in its assimilation.

## Vitamin A

Vitamin A is a very important vitamin for me since I've always had weak eyes. Long before antibiotics came along, doctors and mothers knew of the value of vitamin A in fighting infections, especially respiratory ailments, and they used cod liver oil, which is very high in A. When I was growing up, the only medicines found in our house were aspirin and cod liver oil. Vitamin A is extremely valuable to the defense systems of the body because it helps to keep healthy those parts which come in contact with the invading organisms: the skin, the linings of the respiratory, digestive, and urogenital tracts, and the eyes. Since these are the first line of defense, they must be kept strong. Vitamin A also plays an active role in forming those crucial T and B cells which support the immune system. It is also essential for the development of bone and tooth enamel and is part of the process which forms both red and white corpuscles.

Some nutritionists believe it's better to obtain much of the daily intake of vitamin A from fruits and vegetables in the form of beta-carotene rather than getting it all from fish liver oils. Beta-carotene is converted by the body into a highly potent form of vitamin A. There are a lot to choose from: carrots, collards, mustard greens, kale, spinach, sweet potatoes, papayas, persimmons, and peaches. Any orange fruit or vegetable is high in beta-carotene and many find that making juice from them is an easy way to obtain the daily requirement. That way, nothing gets lost in the cooking process.

Yet, even if you eat a ton of fruits and vegetables, you're still going to come up short, so supplementation is the order of the day. I recommend taking 25,000 units of A per day, which is less than what I take. And when I use my eyes more than usual, as in night driving, I take even more. I realize that A is oil-based and can be stored but I have never read of anyone actually overdosing on the vitamin. The greater problem is obtaining enough to meet the daily needs of the individual.

> YET, EVEN IF YOU EAT A TON OF FRUITS AND VEGETABLES, YOU'RE STILL GOING TO COME UP SHORT, SO SUPPLEMENTATION IS THE ORDER OF THE DAY.

Be sure to take some E and C with your vitamin A supplement because this enhances the curative effect of the A. It's best to take the supplements in balanced doses throughout the day. Most importantly, there has to be some vitamin D present for proper utilization of the A . . . which brings me to the final antioxidant on my list, vitamin D, the current "must-have" supplement on the market.

## Vitamin D

You can't pick up a magazine without seeing a piece on the "sunshine vitamin." It's as if it were just discovered. It's now very much in vogue because so many people are fearful of getting too much sun but don't take a supplement containing any vitamin D, with the result that a great many illnesses have been traced to the lack of this important vitamin.

> FOR EXAMPLE, MEN WITH ADEQUATE LEVELS OF D HAVE ABOUT HALF THE RISK OF HEART ATTACK AS MEN WHO ARE DEFICIENT.

What is actually happening is that people are gulping down loads of vitamin D and neglecting the other antioxidants, A, C, and E, and this doesn't work. Popular magazines, such as *Reader's Digest*, lay down a long list of good things that D does for the body, but fail to add that it is ineffective when taken by itself. Those who read those articles are led to believe that all they need to take to lower their risk of becoming ill is vitamin D in rather large amounts, but that causes problems—it just doesn't work.

Used properly, it's terrific. For example, men with adequate levels of D have about half the risk of heart attack as men who are deficient. Vitamin D also lowers the risk of at least half a dozen types of cancer. Epidemiologist Cedric Garland, M.D. at the University of California, San Diego, believes that if Americans got sufficient amounts of vitamin D, some fifty thousand cases of colorectal cancer could be prevented each year.

Vitamin D is formed by ultraviolet light from sunshine in the oils on the skin, provided you have oils on your skin and they're exposed to sunlight. This would be an excellent source of the vitamin except that most people these days shun sunlight, or wear clothes or live in houses, or the sunlight does not penetrate the thick layer of smog that occurs in many parts of the country.

In addition, even if you do expose your skin to the sun for about 20 to 30 minutes a day, there are other requirements to satisfy before the sunshine is converted to vitamin D. Oil must be present on your skin for this conversion to happen. If you take a shower before going into the sun, the oils are removed and no vitamin D can be formed. Likewise, should you shower or wash your skin immediately after being exposed to the sunlight, the oils are removed and cannot be reabsorbed into the body and no vitamin D makes it into your system. Our parents and grandparents got a sufficient supply of D from the sun because they were outdoors much longer than we are and didn't bathe nearly as often.

An interesting sidebar to this is that during the polio epidemic in the 1940s, it was discovered that children living in the poorer sections of cities caught the disease much less often than those in more prosperous area. The poor kids rarely bathed while the parents of the more affluent scrubbed their kids well to wash off the germs. What they were doing was preventing the children from converting sunshine to vitamin D, which could battle the polio virus.

Of interest to anyone who trains with purpose, vitamin D can greatly improve your energy level. Two minerals, calcium and phosphorus, are energy sources, yet even when they're in sufficient supply, they cannot be utilized unless there is adequate vitamin D present. Phosphorus is a carrier of sugar, transporting it through the intestinal wall and from the bloodstream to be stored as glycogen. Later, before energy can be produced from sugar, the sugar must again combine with phosphorus and this is the case whether the sugar comes directly from the blood or from the breakdown of glycogen. When D is in short supply, the process does not take place. The same is true for calcium because it's so closely linked with phosphorus that what affects one affects the other.

Because of its close ties with the two minerals, vitamin D is essential for strong bones and teeth. In short, it's a valuable vitamin and you need to make sure you're getting a sufficient amount. Be certain you don't buy artificially produced D. It's a waste of money and ineffective. Buy natural products that combine vitamins A and D. As I mentioned, they work in concert, which is why many who have jumped in on the D bandwagon aren't getting the expected results. They're only taking D—and often not the natural variety.

When I wrote in *The Strongest Shall Survive* that I recommended as much as 5,000 units of D per day, I was chastised by many people, most of whom were in the medical profession. They said since D is oil-based and can be stored in the body, I was inviting an overdose with potentially dire consequences. Now, it turns out that most experts agree with me, or rather with Adelle Davis, since that's where I got that figure. If you get ample sunshine, you can get by on less; otherwise, don't be afraid to take that amount every day. I do with no ill effects and with an assurance that I'm supplying my body with all the vitamins and minerals that I need to keep it functioning as I want it to. Or, you can stick with the recommended daily requirements of 200–600 IUs if you wish. But don't be surprised if that low dosage doesn't bring the desired results.

Learn all you can about the various antioxidants and put that knowledge to use. A note in this regard is when you are reading an article in a popular magazine about some antioxidant, consider the source. If that publication carries a ton of ads from pharmaceutical companies, the information is going to be tainted with bias, which is the case with anything on vitamins in *Reader's Digest*. I enjoy the magazine, but I take the pieces on supplements with a grain of salt. Pharmaceutical companies do not promote the usage of natural products to solve medical problems. Since they help to pay the bills with their ads, they have something to say about what's printed in the publication. That's just the way the business operates.

> BUY NATURAL PRODUCTS THAT COMBINE VITAMINS A AND D. AS I MENTIONED, THEY WORK IN CONCERT . . .

Getting stronger and staying physically active and free from illness are completely dependent on knowing how to utilize the various nutritional supplements that are readily available. The antioxidants are your best friends in this ongoing battle.

# Training for Grip Competitions

### David Hurzeler

I have been training my grip specifically for more than 10 years, plus I have organized and competed in many meets in Switzerland, France, and Sweden, and twice in the European Grip Championships, which I won in 2005. The purpose of this article is to share what I have learned over the years about what works and what doesn't in the world of competitive grip.

Grip competitions have become more and more popular recently, with wider media coverage as well as a broader range of athletes coming from different fields, including strongman, powerlifting, climbing, combat sports, and armwrestling. The level of capable athletes has risen fast and it is no longer possible to rely on one's base grip strength and do well in a well-attended all-round grip contest. Along with directly addressing grip strength, specific training for the contest is essential to succeed.

Preparation for a grip contest should ideally be split into two phases: one for overall grip strength improvement, and one for work on specific contest events. Particular care should be taken with hand health, and any injuries should be tackled actively.

> COMPETITIONS ARE WON BY GENERALISTS, NOT BY SPECIALISTS.

### General strength training

First, you should build up the base of the pyramid, clearing up any tweaks and pains you might have, and increasing your general strength to prepare the hands and forearms for the second phase, which will be tougher on the joints.

For this general grip work, a sample of generic grip exercises should be chosen with the following characteristics: simplicity, versatility, comfort, and balance.

Simplicity
Pick exercises that work the area you want to reinforce very directly and which do not need huge amounts of coordination or technique. You do not want to spend too much time getting familiar with the exercise. Also, avoid exercises requiring a high tolerance to pain (like bending). This is not what you are trying to achieve in this phase.

Versatility
Aim for a well-rounded grip program, including crush, support, pinch, and wrist training. Competitions are won by generalists, not by specialists. Also, work both hands and always start with your weaker hand, to give it extra energy and focus.

Comfort
Some of the contest events may well feel uncomfortable to you, but now is not the time to get hurt. In this phase we are looking at sets of 5 to 15 repetitions, so you want to do exercises that feel comfortable enough that you can give them your all. Please note that this refers to biomechanical comfort. As an example, let's look at wrist curls. Some people are very comfortable with a straight bar. For others, a straight bar feels unnatural, and they prefer working with a dumbbell, with the forearm resting on a knee and leaning to the side.

Here are some wrist curl variations you might consider:
- seated, with a straight bar
- seated, with a dumbbell
- seated, with a revolving handle and a low pulley (which has the advantage of offering resistance throughout the whole range of the movement)
- standing, with your hands pronated (double overhand), bar behind the legs (as in a Hack squat)

This last little gem (much favored by the immense Louis Uni, by the way) has many advantages: 1) it allows you to take heavier weights (always a good idea), 2) you can complete forced reps by leaning forward, 3) it provides maximal resistance at the end of the movement, and 4) it works the flexors digitorum, both profundus *and* superficialis (which do not come into play in a flexed-elbow position).

The wrist curl example clearly shows the variations a simple exercise can offer to achieve comfort. Use your imagination and experiment to find ones that feel right to you.

Balance
In this training phase, you definitely want to target any unbalances you might have (which invariably lead to injuries). That means that you are going to work the extensors along with the flexors of the fingers and wrist.

An example of an excellent exercise for correcting these imbalances is the reverse curl on a small diameter bar, with the thumbs on the same side of the bar as the other fingers (IronMind's Eagle Loops also work very well). This exercise offers the advantage—not obvious at first glance—of working both the wrist and the extensors of the fingers. For such hand health-oriented exercises, use longer sets of 15 to 20 reps and aim for a nice forearm burn and pump at the end of the workout.

Grip expert David Horne has shared a generic grip workout, which is perfect example of what we have been talking about:

**Workout to promote balance and hand health:**

1. Two-hands pinch lift for holds (use work gloves to protect your skin).
2. Finger curls with an Olympic bar, overhand grip. Hold it on the last set when you can't do any more finger curls.
3. Two-hand wrist curl with a normal grip and a comfortable range of motion. Do not let the bar slide onto your fingertips like some bodybuilders do. Also, do them with your thumbs under the bar, as you are training your wrists and do not want to fight against the thumbs on top of the bar.
4. Two-hands reverse wrist curl.

# Would you train for a bench press contest only with dumbbells? Of course not.

## Competition preparation—specificity

When getting close to the competition date (the last four weeks, at the very least), it is time to train the exact competition lifts. Would you enter a powerlifting squat meet by doing only front squats? Would you train for a bench press contest only with dumbbells? Of course not. The body needs to adapt to and achieve coordination in the specific events in order to express its full power in those particular exercises. Try to find out what equipment is going to be used and either buy or replicate it as precisely as possible. Again, you would probably not train for a powerlifting squat competition with a safety or cambered bar only, or prepare for a competition requiring a walkout for the squat exclusively in a Monolift.

A crucial factor for grip competitions is the coating of the implements, the feel of their surface. Is the bar going to be knurled? Slick and chromed? Rusty? Seasoned with chalk? Try to find out, and work on that exact surface—you will be amazed at the difference it can make. Some people will use more wrist flexion on a slicker thick bar, for example, so their training will be quite different from that for a rusty bar or a knurled bar, which would perhaps involve more thumb.

Similarly, replicate all the competition conditions you may know about. Are you going to use chalk in powder form or in blocks? What kind of wraps are going to be used for bending? What kind of steel (hot- or cold-rolled), and what diameter and length? How much time are you going to have to warm up? Some of this may seem like very fine tuning, but it will at worst put you in a confident state of mind on the day of the event.

Another thing to consider is the chronology of the competition. If grippers are scheduled to be contested after a thick bar event, for example, you must be prepared for that as your performance will most likely be affected. This does not necessarily mean you should always train grippers after a thick bar—especially if grippers are your weak point, in which case you should, at least some of the time, train grippers first to give them your most. One approach, if for example you decide to devote two days per week to grip workouts, is to train half of the events on day one and the other half on day two. And at least once before the contest, preferably over the last session(s), try doing all the events at sub-max percentages in one workout.

Finally, remember that most grip events are isometric efforts on the forearm muscles, so in this specific contest training phase, you'll want to train isometrically. Full-range moves are no longer what you need unless the event is specifically full-range. Make your

> Try to find out, and work on that exact surface— you will be amazed at the difference it can make.

body learn to work as you will need it to perform on competition day, and don't distract it with general training anymore.

## Prehab and rehab

Hand health and injury
To get the most out of your contest preparation, you must remain injury-free. Never ever skip a warm-up! Hurry one too many times and you might regret it for several days, weeks, or even months if you get unlucky. It is always more tempting to grab a No. 3.5 CoC gripper and squeeze it or to try to bend a spike than it is to try to pick up 600 lb. cold. Not only will you risk injury (and over the long run, probably get one), you will lose energy while not being able to apply full force yet. Treat grip as seriously as you treat back strength. A general body warm-up, such as squats, will work better than a localized hand warm-up.

Again, think balanced agonist–antagonist training during the general grip training phase. Use active recovery between heavy grip workouts if you can. Bring blood to sore muscles and ligaments to accelerate healing and recovery. Use light weights and high reps on simple exercises (such as those used in the first phase), or on specific recovery tools, like David Horne's Orbigrip.

Unfortunately injury is part of sport, and it may happen. If that is the case, first identify the injury. See a doctor and put a name on the pain. You are not going to deal with a sore tendon as you would a broken bone! Once you know exactly what you are facing, try to find alternate pain-free moves that will still allow you to train. Use contrast baths, deep massage, ice, or light pump exercises to bring blood back to the injured area. Pay attention to your nutrition and drink a lot of water.

Hand skin
The skin on your fingers and palms is something to look after closely as well. Calluses may look cool but they are your enemies in grip! Apart from the fact that they do not stick on the implements, they tear, and a ripped callous will probably ruin your competition. Also avoid skin abrasions if you can—they require several days to fully heal and will make you lose time—and find alternatives if you feel your skin is about to give out. For example, train the pinch grip with a towel between your hands and the implement until your skin is back to normal or if you want to do high-rep sets. Two weeks before the competition, do not go all-out on skin-sensitive events: focus on singles and sub-maximal weight which you can control. If calluses start to form, cut them off in a hot bath and possibly use a good moisturizing cream at night on your hands.

Squats
Finally, squat! Squats are your best ally in grip training as they offer the best possible warm-up without taxing your

> TREAT GRIP AS SERIOUSLY AS YOU TREAT BACK STRENGTH.

> SQUATS ARE YOUR BEST ALLY IN GRIP TRAINING . . .

grip at all. Test yourself on grippers after or before a squat workout, and you will feel the magic of squats.

Without getting into too much detail, as this is not our purpose here, squats enhance general body strength and activation of the body's nervous system; they help you handle big weights in heavy grip events; and they have an indirect effect on your grip as well. And lastly, squats help with recovery.

Find a form of squatting which suits you well. Beware of low-bar squats if these hurt your shoulders, as this will also affect your grip workouts. I find high-bar full back squats to be what I need, but you'll want to experiment with other kinds, like safety, Manta Ray, or front squats.

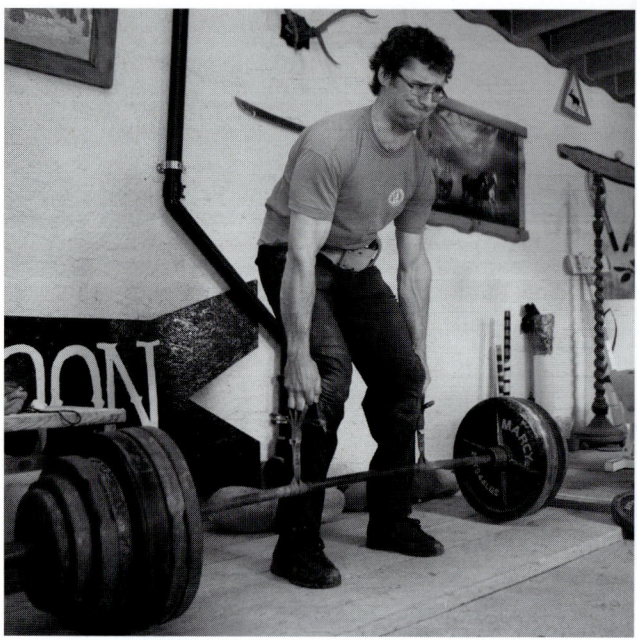

David Hurzeler warms up before lifting 280 kg in the 2-finger-per-hand Eagle Loops deadlift event at a recent Swiss grip competition.
Muriel Antille photo.

### Have fun

To conclude, do not forget to enjoy yourself! During the first phase at least, find exercises you enjoy, or offer yourself from time to time a "pleasure" workout that includes all your favorite grip events, as long as you are not taking any unnecessary risks. This will boost both your motivation and confidence, as we tend to be better at what we like—and without pleasure, your drive will eventually disappear. Similarly, if you are lucky enough to have a training partner, challenge each

> FINALLY, DO NOT DREAD THE COMPETITION—LOOK FORWARD TO IT!

other now and again in friendly grip bouts. Do not do this at every workout but once in a while, and it will add that extra spice to your training.

Finally, do not dread the competition—look forward to it! You will always learn something new at a competition, be it about yourself, about a new exercise or technique, or about the other competitors. Plus, grip competitions are a ton of fun and in most cases very friendly, so if you haven't one in your sights, find one now. **M**

# The Search for
# Harold Wood

**Roger Davis**

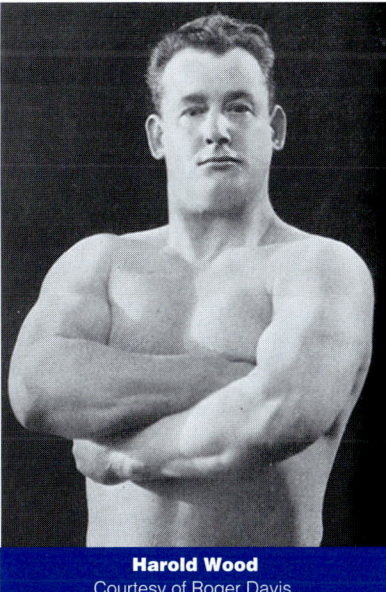

**Harold Wood**
Courtesy of Roger Davis.

My search for Harold Wood began one lazy Sunday afternoon as I was browsing through some old magazines that are part of my collection of early weightlifting history literature. The particular area under my review was a list of all the British amateur weightlifting champions from the period 1911 to 1937, a Golden Age for British weightlifting, with a pool of 42 different lifts to choose from for the championships. This was long before the press, snatch, and clean and jerk were selected to be used solely in the Olympic Games. What interested me greatly was that one name was dominant in the heavyweight division, with victories in 1912, and then 1924 through 1929, a virtually unbroken reign of some 17 years at the top. Even though I had come across the name on several occasions, I could not recall one single comprehensive history of Harold Wood, the heavyweight champion for all that time. I wanted to find out more . . . the search had begun.

I began with a 1932 edition of the book *Weight-Lifting Made Easy and Interesting*, written by W. A. Pullum, the man who almost single-handedly transformed weightlifting from a circus and theatre act into a modern sport. A brief history of his most successful pupils included Harold Wood of Battersea, along with a photo of a large and muscular man and a short summary of his greatest lifts throughout his career.

The *Health and Strength* annual of 1929 listed all of the British records at that time, and it was with some surprise that I saw that 19 of the possible records in the heavyweight division were owned by Harold Wood.

Now I had begun to make a connection. As a competitive weightlifter myself, I could relate to the weights that had been lifted: very good lifts for the period, and far superior to the average man's strength (both now and then), but weights that are eclipsed in

| British records held by Harold Wood in 1929 | |
| --- | --- |
| Right-hand military press | 103.75 lb. |
| Left-hand military press | 110.00 |
| Right-hand snatch | 156.25 |
| Left-hand dumbbell swing | 170.50 |
| Pullover and press | 311.25 |
| Pullover and push | 387.75 |
| Two-hands dumbbells swing | 170.25 |
| Two-hands dumbbells press | 200.00 |
| Two-hands dumbbells push | 213.75 |
| Two-hands dumbbells clean & jerk | 237.75 |
| Two-hands dumbbells continental jerk | 238.25 |
| Two-hands dumbbells anyhow | 250.50 |
| Barbell military press | 216.50 |
| Barbell push | 254.25 |
| Snatch | 212.00 |
| Press behind neck | 193.00 |
| Jerk behind neck | 275.00 |
| Clean and jerk | 287.75 |
| Deadlift | 539.50 |

today's modern competitive arena with professional athletes, coaches, top-of-the-line equipment, nutrition, and dare I say it, performance-enhancing drugs. Harold came before all this, when the sport was still a working man's hobby and in a developmental stage, when lifters grafted a full day before attending the gym.

A small article in the 1974 *Anvils, Horseshoes and Cannons: The History of Strongmen* by Leo Gaudreau included a brief account of some of Harold's strength feats and the fact that he represented Britain in the Olympics (I later found out this was in 1924 and 1928 where he placed 17th and 13th, respectively), as well as a few anecdotes. One was an interesting account of the time Harold met the world famous strongman performer "Samson," whose real name was Alexander Zass, at an exhibition at the Camberwell Weight Lifting Club. As part of his regular act, Zass challenged anyone in the audience to punch him as hard as possible in the stomach, a feat that had been tried by many boxers of the time with little reaction from Samson. Harold was pushed onto the stage by his followers and expressed concern that he didn't wish to hurt the man before him. Upon being reassured by Samson, Harold let loose a mighty blow, and although Samson stayed upright, he turned pale and staggered back six feet. Upon recovering he admitted it was the hardest punch he had ever taken, and this was from someone the author describes as a hard-living man, taking no care of himself and content to believe that an iron constitution would see him through whatever he did.

A phone call to strength journal collector David Horne furnished me with a 1952 *Health and Strength* magazine with a small article on Harold Wood by W. A. Pullum, and the information it contained proved priceless to my research. First and most importantly, Harold's birth name was actually Kirwood. Why he had changed this I could not imagine, but this information would be essential when investigating his birth and death records. Other details that filled in the gaps were his upbringing by an uncle in Yorkshire in a hard and sparse environment, and his interest in gymnastics and acrobatics from ages 10 to 20, at which time he was introduced to weightlifting by the renowned Swiss weightlifter Albert Soguel.

Pullum's article noted that at his first competition in 1912 Harold won the 12-stone class before making a permanent

> . . . HAROLD LET LOOSE A MIGHTY BLOW, AND ALTHOUGH SAMSON STAYED UPRIGHT HE TURNED PALE AND STAGGERED BACK SIX FEET.

> MY HEAD SPUN. THE ONLY POSSIBLE EXPLANATION WAS THAT HAROLD HAD GOTTEN BLIND DRUNK, FELL, AND FROZE TO DEATH ON THAT COLD JANUARY NIGHT.

move into the heavies. The Great War put Harold's lifting on hold, but he proved himself on another platform with many knockout wins in army boxing competitions (this sheds light on the Samson punch!). After a brief summary of his lifting career, the article explained that Harold suffered from gout in his later competitive years but continued to lift to encourage his nemesis Ron Walker. A final comment on Harold's trip up from the country to visit Pullum, presumably in the 1950s, described him as being in great shape and virile and forceful as ever.

Armed with this data I went to the family records office in Islington to try to obtain his birth and death certificates—the office is an amazing place, with row after row of books containing all the births, marriages, and deaths in Britain since records began. I managed to locate and order certificates for Harold Montague Kirwood, born 18 January 1889, died 25 January 1954 at Standon, Hertfordshire. His place of death interested me greatly as Standon is a mere 20 miles from my home location, and I waited the five days with eager anticipation until the full details could be received.

I received the details early on a Monday morning whilst leaving for work and couldn't resist opening the documents whilst sitting in a slow-moving traffic jam. The birth certificate gave details that I expected and a specific birth address of 38 Redburn Street, Chelsea. The death certificate was more surprising, noting his place of death outside his house Wellfields, Wellpond Green, Standon, Ware. The cause of death was extreme cold, alcohol and misadventure.

My head spun. The only possible explanation was that Harold had gotten blind drunk, fell, and froze to death on that cold January night. It was a shock; I felt saddened and slightly disappointed that this great lifter's life had ended in such a tragic way. Like most modern-day people I expect my chosen heroes to be whiter than white, with no thought to the complexities of their lives.

A trip out to the delightful village of Wellpond Green proved fruitless in locating a house named Wellfields; still, I was aware that house owners may change house names as they see fit, and I decided I needed to find some village archives for the original name. As I left the village I mused that the working-class boy from Battersea had done rather well for himself (especially as his death certificate described his occupation as "rat catcher") to find himself in such a now prosperous and delightful setting.

A few days later it occurred to me that some of the older residents of the village might still remember Harold and have further information for me, so I phoned the source of all local information, the village pub. The Nag's Head pub had a very friendly and interested landlord, who put me in contact with a gentleman who had been in the village since boyhood and had just contributed to a book on the area. Unfortunately he could not recall Harold, and had never heard of Wellfields.

A last-ditch attempt to identify the house found me at the Standon parish records where two very helpful ladies rang around local residents for further information. My heart sank as I heard that a local 92-year-old had just passed away, and he would certainly have known Harold. Two more calls, no success. Then I heard, "Oh, you did know him, great, and you can come down, see you soon." That was how I was introduced to Gordon Wheeler, a delightful gentleman with a warm smile whose family had been the village bakers during those years. "Yes, I remember Harold" he said, "I used to deliver my bread to him as a boy, a great big bloke he was, used to have a great leather belt to keep his stomach in." Could that have been his old lifting belt? Harold had obviously continued to let his weight grow, in stark contrast to the description by W. A. Pullum, who obviously wanted to present the good health of one of his former pupils for business reasons.

The mystery of Wellfields was cleared up when Gordon explained that "Harold lived in an old railway carriage in a farmer's field; he kept pigs and goats and scraped a living. Nice bloke he was, though, very friendly. He had daughters living with him, they moved there about 1943 to get away from the Blitz in London, lovely looking girls they were," he said with a glint in his eye.

Gordon generously took me to the location where the railway carriage used to be, halfway down Blind Lane. The field is overgrown now, but in my mind's eye I could see the railway carriage and a portly Harold standing outside. I thanked Gordon and then drove to the beautiful church of St. Mary's at Standon on a hunch. As I entered, the resident vicar Rev. David Humphrey was in the final stages of preparing for a funeral. He met my enquiries with great enthusiasm and let me peruse the church records, where I found a 1954 entry for Harold Kirwood. A study of the graveyard plans located the grave for me, and as I climbed the slippery route to the top of the churchyard, my heart was beating fast; I wondered what his epitaph would say, and what family details would be revealed. I stopped, checked my location—a beautiful spot overlooking the village—and then with a dawning realisation found myself looking at an unmarked grave. What else would you expect for a rat catcher?

> . . . MY HEART WAS BEATING FAST; I WONDERED WHAT HIS EPITAPH WOULD SAY, AND WHAT FAMILY DETAILS WOULD BE REVEALED.

As a fellow weightlifter and open-minded in religious matters, I muttered a few words of greeting to Harold, and sheepishly left the spot. My final appointment of the day was at the County Hall where I studied microfiche of the local papers of the day. After some time I found a one-column article on the unfortunate circumstance concerning Harold's death. Indeed drink had been involved, a bottle of vodka drunk with a friend, a lift home, a fall, and then the startling finding of Harold's body the next morning. I found no obituary, no report on his funeral or attendees there; the only link with his weightlifting past was the local policeman describing him as a "very strong man."

I got the distinct impression that Harold had kept his previous weightlifting feats unknown to his new neighbours. What had happened to the countless medals and trophies that he had accumulated I could only surmise,

> HE OBVIOUSLY STILL LOVED HIS LIFTING, AND I COULD RELATE TO THAT PASSION.

although I now have the good fortune to have two of Harold's medals as pride of place in my collection, finds on eBay. Why the weightlifting fraternity had failed to erect a suitable headstone I could not understand; still, time moves on and fame, however great, is short-lived.

Two further connections were made. I have in the past had the good fortune of training with Wally Pullum (nephew of W. A. Pullum), who told me that he was trained by Jim Franklin of Battersea, who was in turn trained by Harold Wood, so indirectly Harold has had an influence on my lifting—I found that pleasant to think on. Another communication with David Horne provided me with full details of all the BAWLA Olympic champions from 1932 to 1937. As the Pullum article had hinted, Harold was still there, coming second to Ron Walker each year approaching his fifties, still lifting and in some cases achieving personal bests, including a 310-lb. continental clean and jerk in 1932. He obviously still loved his lifting, and I could relate to that passion.

This is about the end of my research. I have tried to contact remaining family members, and have checked electoral registers and made directory enquiries, and even though the Kirwood name is very rare, I have had no luck. Harold's daughters would probably have changed their maiden names some time ago.

As I try to make sense of all this data, I am trying to understand the man that I have been searching for this period of time, but realise I will never know the full extent of his life. With my typical modern and pampered life, how can I understand a man born into a working-class family in Victorian London, who survived the Great War and then the Depression, and who was driven into the countryside by the Second World War to support himself and his family long before adequate social support was available? Yes, he was a big drinker, as were most people of that time, and who could blame him?

A final finding was a description of Harold's 1928 pullover and push record of 387 lb. It relates how Harold sipped from a quart bottle of beer between attempts, but when the record was finally achieved, the crowd went wild, as Harold was "greatly loved" within the weightlifting community. This ties in with Wally Pullum's expression of sadness at the news of Harold's death and his statement, "I liked Harold Wood very much and as I have said before, so did a lot of other people. When a man's passing is regretted by so many, such regard constitutes the best tribute to his true character and its values."

My lasting connection with Harold is and always will be love of the weights. As I load up the barbell to 310 lb. and acknowledge the strength required to put this overhead, I can think of the only epitaph that seems suitable to the occasion: "Harold Wood, 1889–1954, A Strong Man."

# Metabolic Conditioning

**Brian Mangravite**

It is typically accepted as fact that physical condition falls into one of two categories: muscular strength or cardiovascular ability. It is usually considered a fact that the two are mutually exclusive—you do certain activities to produce cardiovascular fitness, which produce little or no improvements in strength, and other activities to produce muscular strength, which result in little or no improvement in cardiovascular fitness.

There is some truth to those assessments. Very low-resistance movements carried out for a prolonged period of time result in improved cardiovascular ability. That kind of activity—very low intensity coupled almost invariably with overuse of the muscles involved—is pretty much guaranteed to not improve muscular strength. In fact, not infrequently such exercise results in losses of muscular strength.

Conversely, high-resistance movements done relatively briefly and intensely (even high-rep movements rarely last more than a couple of minutes) result in increased strength but are not known for more than relatively modest improvements in cardiovascular ability.

When an athlete exhibits both cardiovascular ability and great muscular strength at the same time, those states are usually attained by the use of two different training protocols—aerobic conditioning and high-resistance training. Generally speaking, an athlete can work very hard for a brief period of time; or he can work at a very low level of intensity for a prolonged period of time. But he can't work very hard for a very long time.

Or can he?

Arthur Jones postulated a third form of conditioning, called "metabolic conditioning," during a large-scale research program at West Point, the United States military academy, using 100 cadets over a six-week period. One of the things Jones set out to test was to what degree cardiovascular ability could be improved in a strength-building regimen with no aerobic training involved. He had representatives there from the Cooper Aerobic Institute to perform the before and after tests to remove any doubts about the results. Reportedly, when these representatives showed the results to Dr. Kenneth Cooper, he refused to believe them—he ordered his own people out of his office and threw the reports in the garbage. You see, in six weeks, the test subjects had a 60% increase in strength—which is an amazing result—and also an equivalent increase in aerobic capacity. Without doing any aerobic training for six weeks, the test subjects decreased their two-mile run time by an average of 88 seconds. The control group, which ran for aerobic training, improved by an average of only 20 seconds. By this measure, the test group improved by more than four-fold—without doing any conventional aerobic training—over the control group.

What can be translated from these results is that it is neither necessary nor desirable to follow two separate kinds of training to accomplish cardiovascular fitness and muscular strength. High levels of both can be achieved with the same protocol.

As interesting as these results are, it was the discovery of that third, previously undefined, element of fitness that Jones called metabolic conditioning that is most exciting. One can only achieve metabolic conditioning through training with that combined, West Point experiment-style of training: the ability to work at a high level of intensity (close to 100%) for twenty or more minutes straight. You can't work an individual muscle group for that long, that's impossible; but you can work the entire body for that long. Workouts consist of 12 to 15 exercises done for 1 set each. Each set is carried to the point of absolute failure after a minimum of 7 and up to a maximum of 12 reps, with no rest between sets. You don't rush the sets—the exercises need to be executed with proper form—but you do rush between sets from one exercise to the next.

> WITHOUT DOING ANY AEROBIC TRAINING FOR SIX WEEKS, THE TEST SUBJECTS DECREASED THEIR TWO-MILE RUN TIME BY AN AVERAGE OF 88 SECONDS.

Interestingly, although the test subjects performed three workouts per week, they only performed one of those workouts in the non-stop, no-rest fashion. For the other workouts they were permitted brief rests, although Jones doesn't state how long they were allowed to rest. It was probably not long, as Jones traditionally pushed trainees pretty hard.

It should also be stated that there needs to be a breaking-in period at the start of this kind of training. Push someone into this kind of training too quickly and "it will literally make people sick, immediately sick, sick to the point of vomiting and then passing out" (Jones). When starting this program, you need to allow a couple of minutes between sets, gradually reducing the rest time between each set. The goal is to eventually reach zero rest between sets for one of the workouts each week.

Some critics might argue that this metabolic conditioning is nothing more than strength coupled with aerobic capacity training. By most standards, the cadets in the West Point experiment were already pretty highly conditioned; they were experienced weight trainers who also trained aerobically. Yet several of

> PUSH SOMEONE INTO THIS KIND OF TRAINING TOO QUICKLY AND "IT WILL LITERALLY MAKE PEOPLE SICK, IMMEDIATELY SICK, SICK TO THE POINT OF VOMITING AND THEN PASSING OUT." (JONES)

the subjects, as mentioned earlier, when launched into this training a bit too rapidly, literally collapsed. They actually showed signs of impending shock—they were completely unable to continue. Respiration was not overly stressed. Heart rate was elevated, but not excessively. Muscle groups were being taxed sequentially—in other words, legs were stressed before different torso groups—so it wasn't muscular failure causing the collapse. The subjects were simply unable to continue.

Jones recounts that forcing them to continue would undoubtedly have caused them to go into shock. After five or six break-in workouts, however, those same subjects were able to complete the workouts without stopping. Something changed. Some element of conditioning improved to the point where a work level previously impossible became possible. What was the change? Jones theorized, and he readily admitted that he had no evidence to support it, that the metabolic processes that convert fuel into available energy to drive the body through these workouts became more efficient, hence his term "metabolic conditioning."

> COACHES, WHAT DO YOU THINK WOULD HAPPEN TO THE OPPOSITION IF YOUR TEAM NEVER HAD TO HUDDLE?

What does this mean to the athlete? To a powerlifter or an Olympic lifter, probably not much. But in any sport where there is an advantage to producing peak, or near peak, power output for a prolonged period, this is revolutionary. Wrestling and MMA; military and law enforcement; elite forces like SEALs, Rangers, and SWAT teams—all will benefit from this type of training. How about football? Coaches, what do you think would happen to the opposition if your team never had to huddle? If the opposing team never got the chance for even a few seconds of rest because your team went back to the play without a pause and showed no loss of strength or ability due to fatigue?

Metabolic conditioning is an amazing development in the area of physical conditioning; unfortunately, it has been underutilized. Don't make the same mistake. If you could use superhuman strength and endurance at the same time, give these techniques a try. M

Go to arthurjonesexercise.com for a complete compilation of Arthur Jones's writings assembled by Brian D. Johnston.

**2010 dotFit World Strongman Super Series Mohegan Sun Grand Prix:**

# Local Cop Locks Up the Win—Again

**Randall J. Strossen, Ph.D.**
Publisher & Editor-in-chief

The Mohegan Sun combines a top drawer casino and hotel with excellent restaurants and high street shopping, plus world-class entertainment; and while all of that is nothing to sneeze at, what really distinguishes the Mohegan Sun is the people who work there. To a person, the staff is friendly, helpful, and knowledgeable. Summing up the situation, dotFit COO Odd Haugen pointed out that it's the same people year after year, "which really tells you something about the place."

Haugen should know because it was his group that first brought strongman to the Mohegan Sun in 2005, where the fit for strongman was quickly recognized by Mohegan Sun Sports and Entertainment Director Bob Yalen, whose background includes stints at ESPN and ABC Sports and whose honors include winning three Sports Emmys.

Derek Poundstone made it three in a row at the 2010 Mohegan Sun—does he own this place or what?

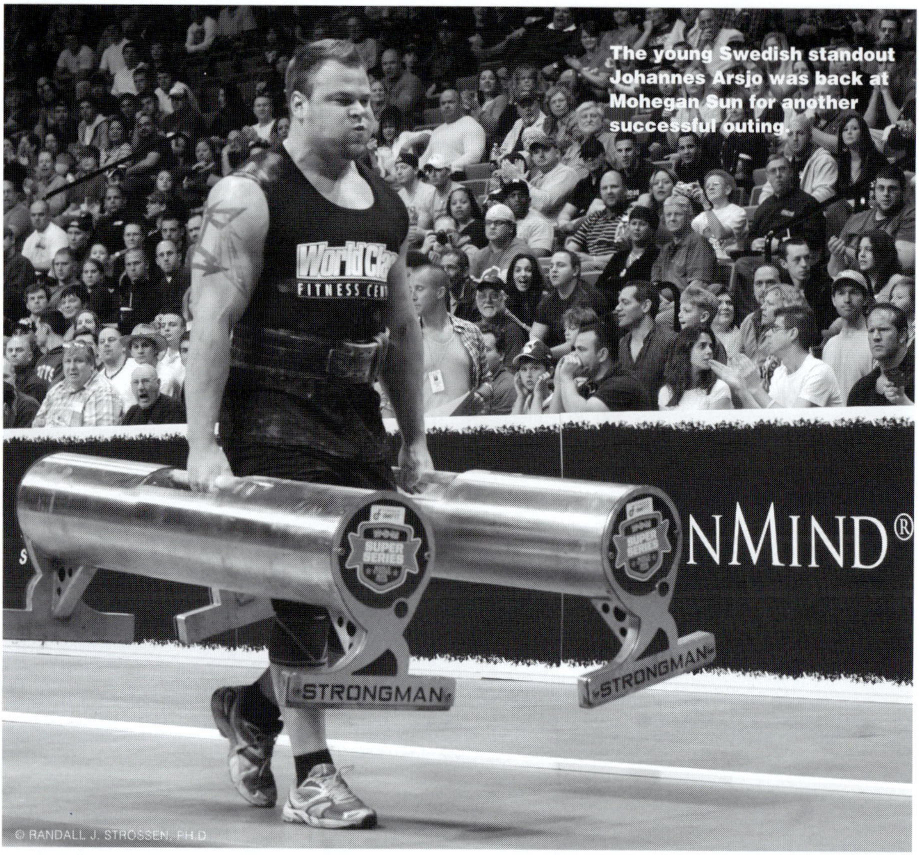

The young Swedish standout Johannes Arsjo was back at Mohegan Sun for another successful outing.

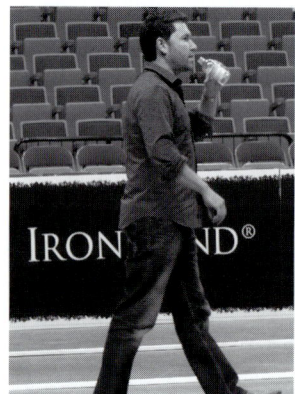

Andy Quinn, who produced and directed the TV show, walks the set before the cameras roll.

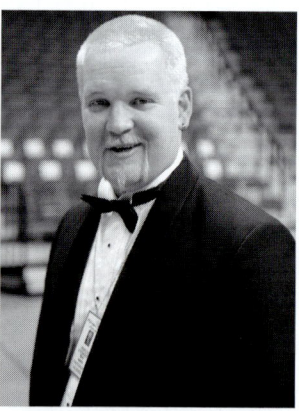

Looking spiffy in his tuxedo (a good cigar not far away), Sweden's Anders Axklo was the TV/broadcast emcee.

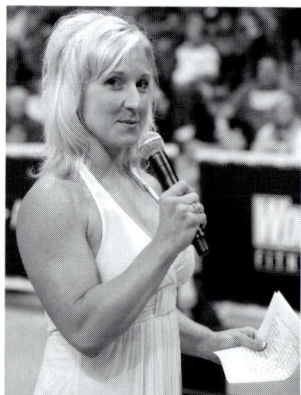

Callie ("I'm not camera shy") Best did the honors as the live audience emcee.

All photos by Randall J. Strossen.

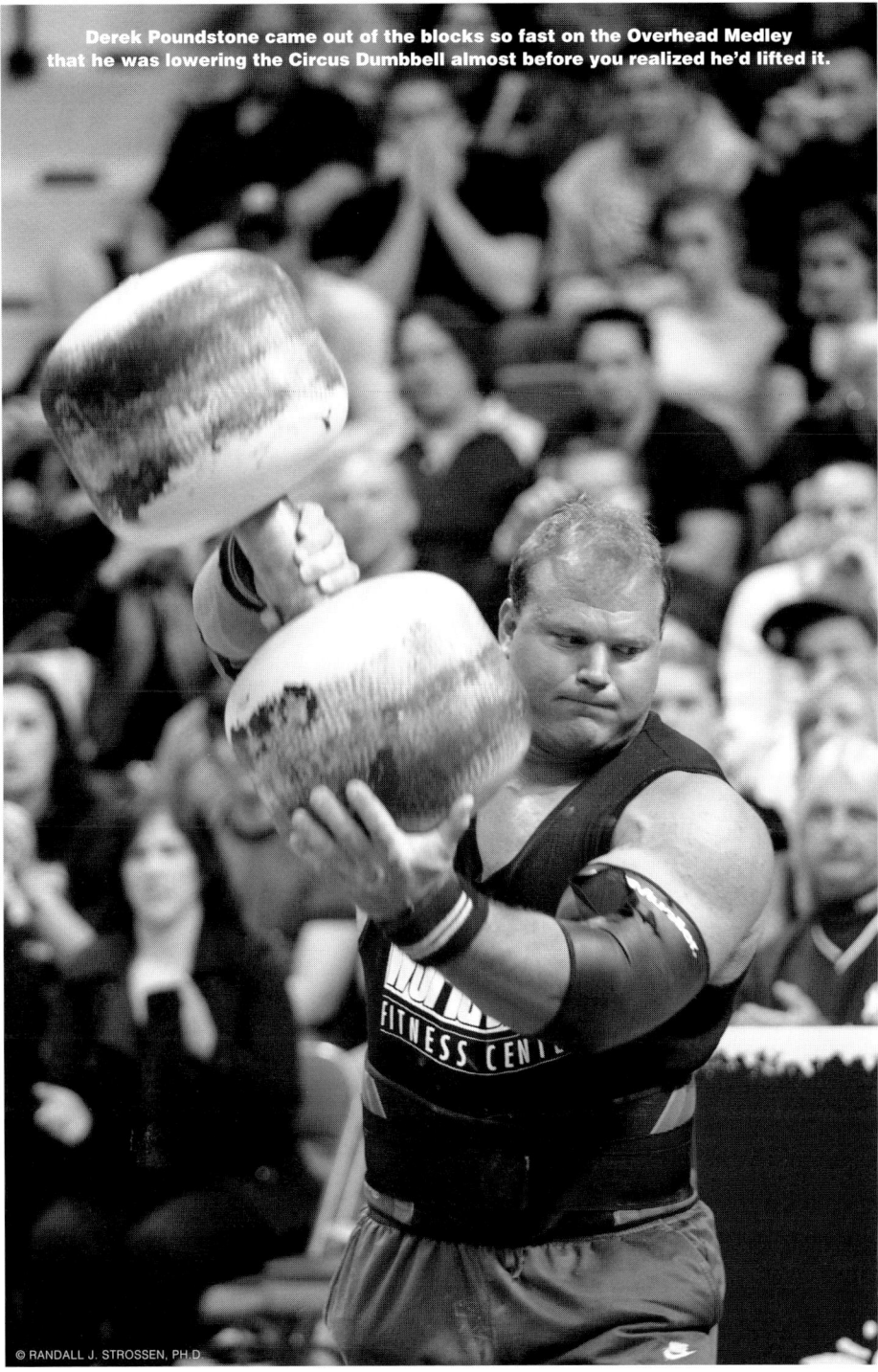
Derek Poundstone came out of the blocks so fast on the Overhead Medley that he was lowering the Circus Dumbbell almost before you realized he'd lifted it.

No need for him to jerk world record level weights on the Apollon's Axle—Derek Poundstone just presses them.

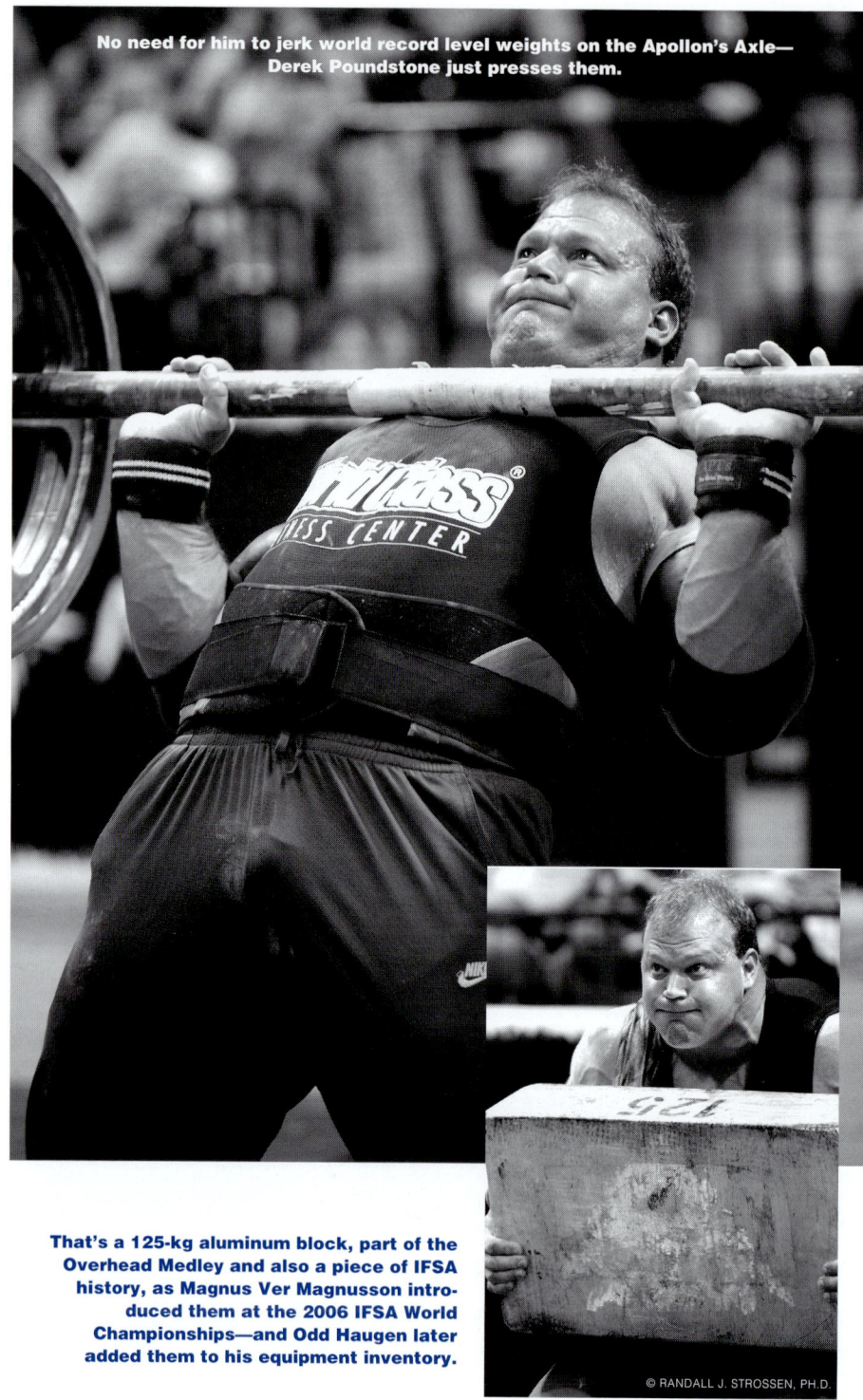

That's a 125-kg aluminum block, part of the Overhead Medley and also a piece of IFSA history, as Magnus Ver Magnusson introduced them at the 2006 IFSA World Championships—and Odd Haugen later added them to his equipment inventory.

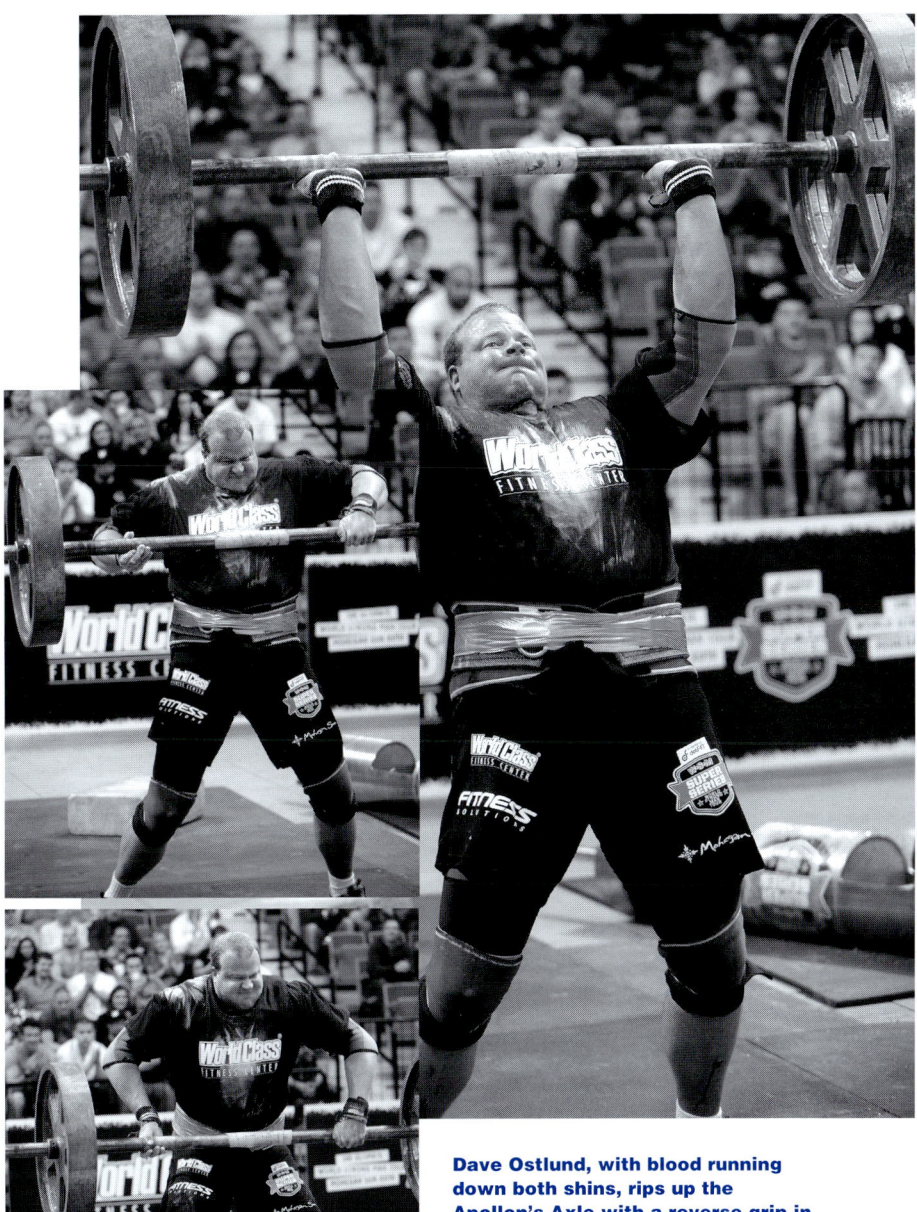

Dave Ostlund, with blood running down both shins, rips up the Apollon's Axle with a reverse grip in the Overhead Medley, and once he got it to his shoulders, he just lay back and pressed it overhead.

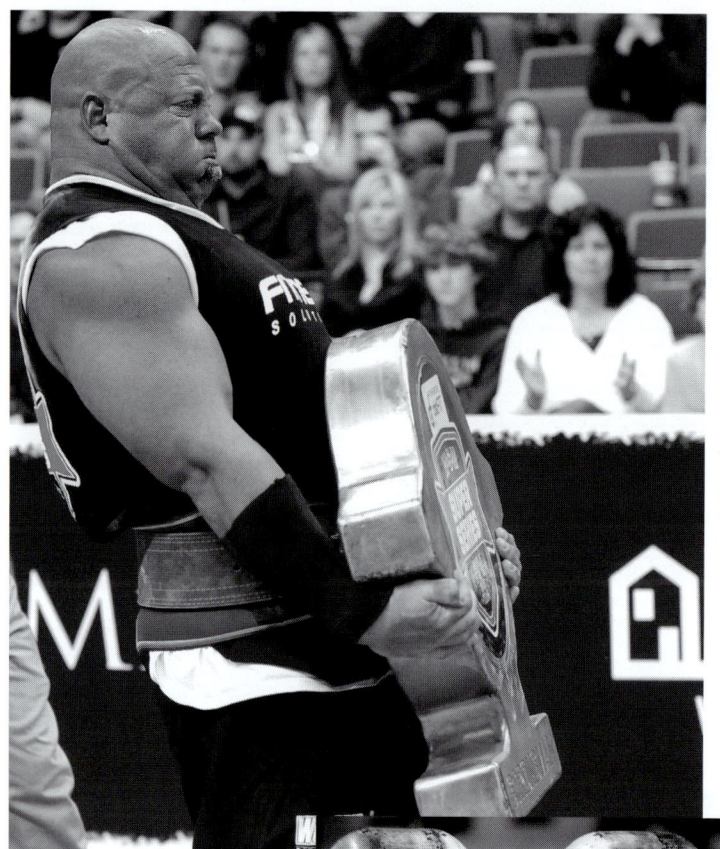

With the Shield hanging low, Nick Best fought for each inch. Later he said that the extra effort was for his then fiancée and now wife, Callie.

Louis-Philippe Jean, the young Quebec strongman who made a name for himself with his prowess on the dumbbells at Fortissimus 2008, gives the Circus Dumbbell a quick ride up.

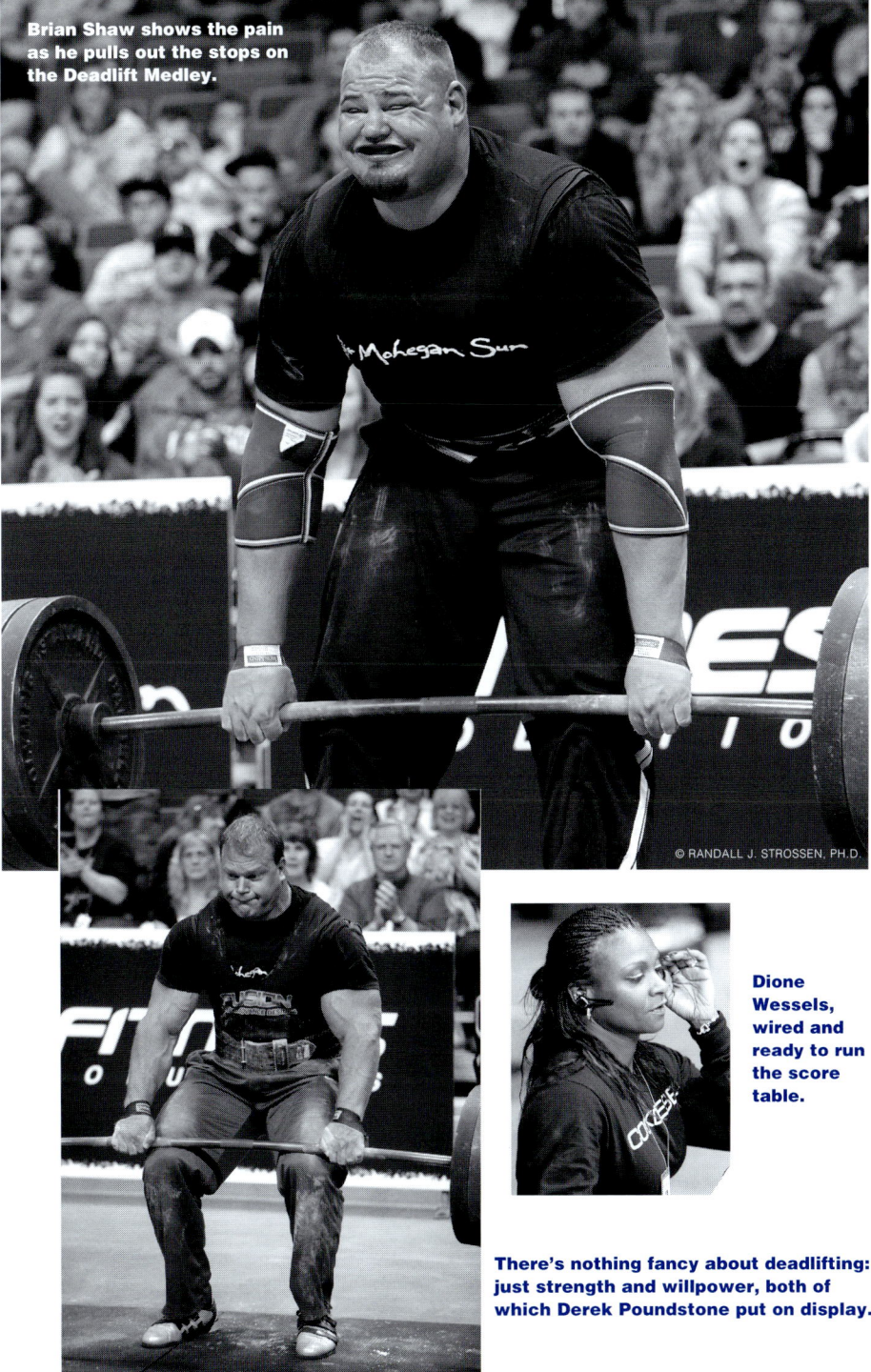

Brian Shaw shows the pain as he pulls out the stops on the Deadlift Medley.

Dione Wessels, wired and ready to run the score table.

There's nothing fancy about deadlifting: just strength and willpower, both of which Derek Poundstone put on display.

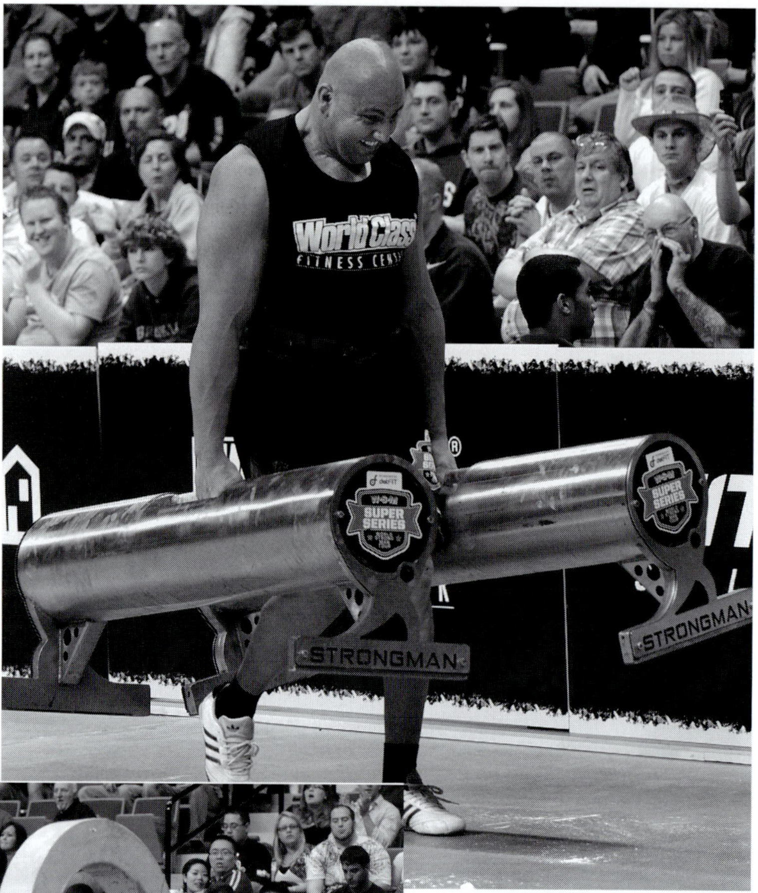

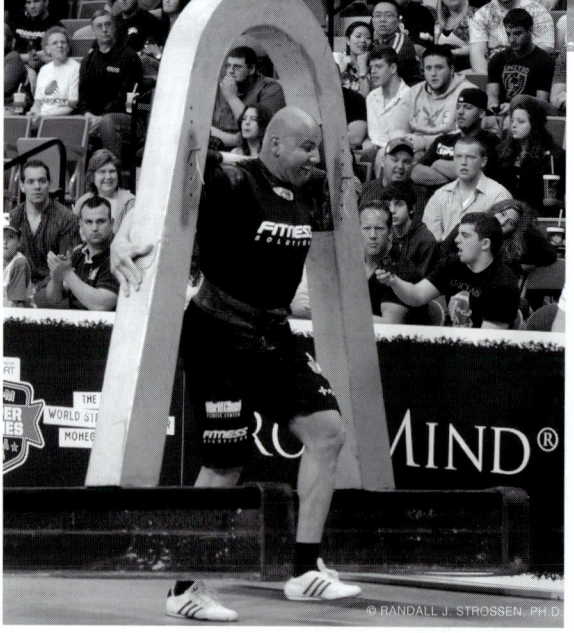
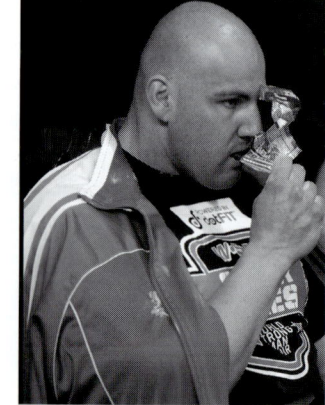

Is carbo loading the secret of Stojan Todorchev's fleet feet? If Derek Poundstone had had a radar gun with him, he might have had to write up Stojan for speeding.

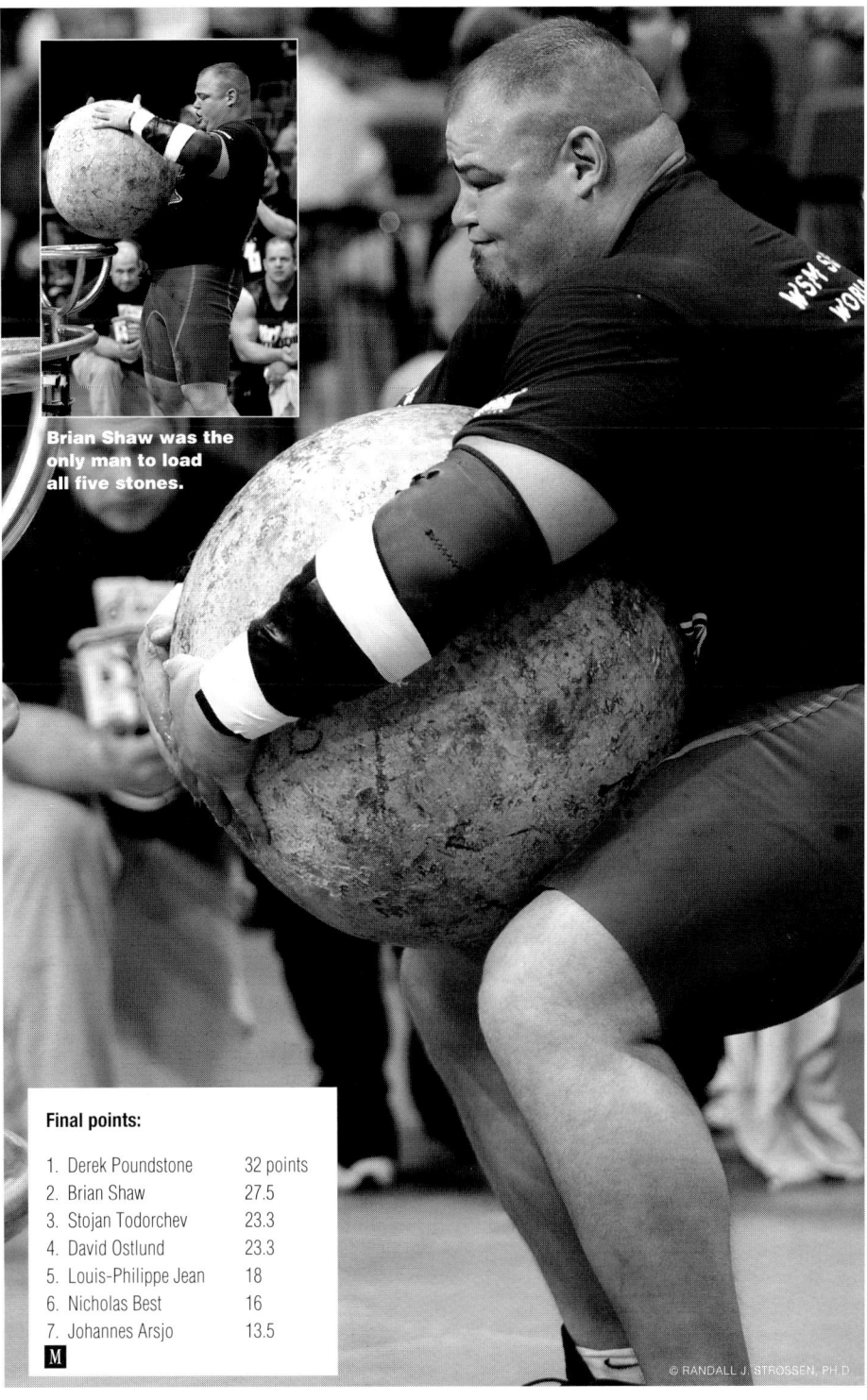

Brian Shaw was the only man to load all five stones.

**Final points:**

1. Derek Poundstone — 32 points
2. Brian Shaw — 27.5
3. Stojan Todorchev — 23.3
4. David Ostlund — 23.3
5. Louis-Philippe Jean — 18
6. Nicholas Best — 16
7. Johannes Arsjo — 13.5

# Pudzianowski or Savickas:

## Who is the Greatest All-Time Strongman?

### M. Andrew Holowchak, Ph.D.

Mariusz Pudzianowski of Poland is perhaps the most recognizable figure in the history of the sport of strongman. He has dominated the World's Strongest Man (WSM) competitions since the turn of the century. Except for 2001 when he did not compete, he has battled for the title in every WSM since 2000, and impressively has won five times (2002, 2003, 2005, 2007, and 2008) and placed second twice (2006 and 2009). Many think that Pudzianowski's dominance in WSM competitions hands down makes him the greatest strongman since the turn of the century, if not of all time.

Lesser known but equally as impressive as Pudzianowski is Lithuania's Zydrunas Savickas. Savickas has won two out of three International Federation of Strength Athletes (IFSA) world titles (2004 and 2005) and the Fortissimus Strength Challenge (FSC) in 2009, and he won the Arnold Strongman Classic (ASC) in six straight attempts (2003 to 2008). He has also recently claimed his first WSM title [2009], after having come in second on three occasions. In claiming those various titles, he has broken numerous world records in major strongman events. Many think that Savickas's capture of four significant titles gives him a more speckled dossier and makes him the greatest strongman since the turn of the century, if not of all time.

Who really is the better strongman of the two?

### The case for Pudzianowski

Pudzianowski is a physically outstanding specimen. At 6' 1" tall and around 310 lb., he is massively muscled and superbly conditioned and carries little bodyfat.

Pudzianowski is also one of the most tenacious competitors that WSM has ever seen. One of his biggest accomplishments was taking the WSM title in 2007 after he had narrowly lost it to Phil Pfister by a couple of seconds in the Atlas Stones in 2006. In 2007, he took two first places and four second places in seven events to win the title. Most impressive was his improvement in the Fingal's Fingers event, where he went from sixth in 2006 to second in 2007.

> MANY THINK THAT PUDZIANOWSKI'S DOMINANCE IN WSM COMPETITIONS HANDS DOWN MAKES HIM HE GREATEST STRONGMAN SINCE . . .

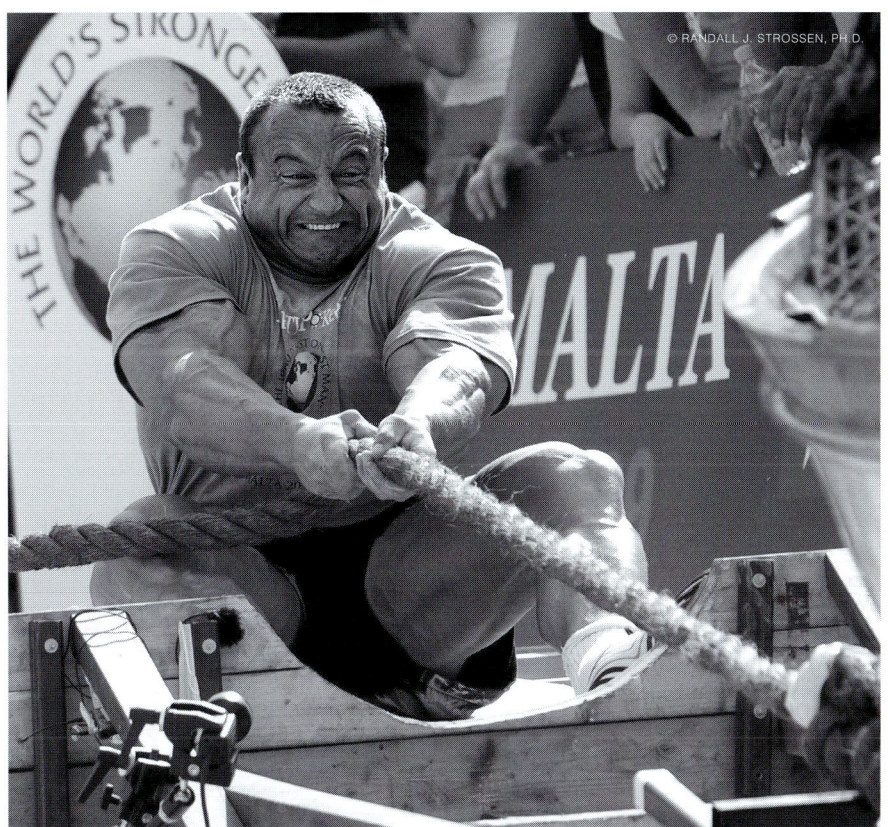

**The Boat Pull at the 2009 World's Strongest Man contest once again showcased the competitiveness of Mariusz Pudzianowski.**

Pudzianowski is also perhaps the most focused strongman that WSM has ever seen. He has an uncanny capacity to eliminate potential distractions and focus on each event to the exclusion of others. His mechanical efficiency in events speaks to his extraordinary mental preparation. In moving events, like the Power Stairs and the Medley, he is especially difficult to beat.

Pudzianowski's résumé of major strongman competitions may be summed as follows:

### Pudzianowski's placings

|      | WSM | IFSA | ASC | FSC |
|------|-----|------|-----|-----|
| 2002 | 1   |      |     |     |
| 2003 | 1   |      | 4   |     |
| 2004 | 3*  | —    | 5   |     |
| 2005 | 1   | —    | —   |     |
| 2006 | 2   | —    | 6   |     |
| 2007 | 1   |      | —   |     |
| 2008 | 1   |      | —   | —   |
| 2009 | 2   |      | —   | —   |

**Key**
—     did not compete
(blank)     lack of competition/federation that year
*     disqualification due to performance-enhancing substances

All photos by Randall J. Strossen.

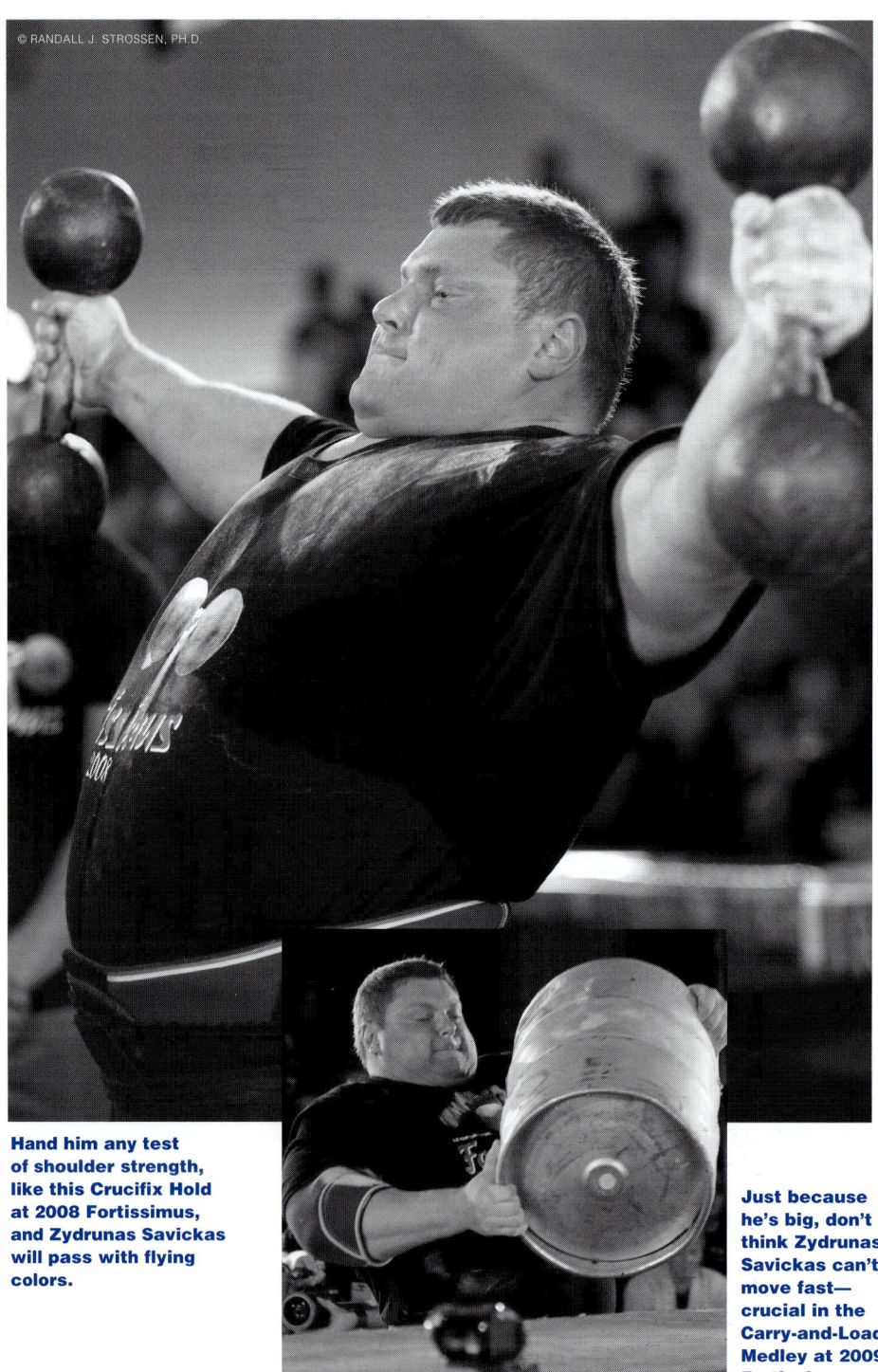

Hand him any test of shoulder strength, like this Crucifix Hold at 2008 Fortissimus, and Zydrunas Savickas will pass with flying colors.

Just because he's big, don't think Zydrunas Savickas can't move fast—crucial in the Carry-and-Load Medley at 2009 Fortissimus.

## The case for Savickas

Savickas, in contrast to Pudzianowski, is not as physically impressive. To those not initiated in strength sports, he looks more like a sumo wrestler than a strongman, yet he is extraordinarily massive. At 6' 3" in height, he often competes at a weight that nears 400 lb.

Appearances notwithstanding, Savickas is a serious, dominant strongman. He has won an extraordinary number of strongman titles and has placed first in IFSA, ASC, FSC, and most recently WSM competitions. He is the holder of numerous strongman world records in significant strongman events. For instance, he has pressed overhead 468 lb. at the 2009 European Log Press Championships and has pulled 1,016 lb. in the Hummer Tire Deadlift at the ASC in 2008. His best powerlifts are 936 lb. in the squat, 628 lb. in the bench press (raw), and 897 lb. in the deadlift.

Savickas's résumé of major strongman competitions may be summed up below:

### Savickas's placings

|      | WSM | IFSA | ASC | FSC |
|------|-----|------|-----|-----|
| 2002 | 2   | —    |     |     |
| 2003 | 2   |      | 1   |     |
| 2004 | 2   | 1    | 1   |     |
| 2005 | —   | 1    | 1   |     |
| 2006 | —   | 2    | 1   |     |
| 2007 | —   |      | 1   |     |
| 2008 | —   |      | 1   | 2   |
| 2009 | 1   |      | —   | 1   |

## Head-to-head comparison

Each strongman has an impressive résumé, so how is one to decide between them? Who is the real strongest man in the world—Pudzianowski or Savickas?

From 2004 to 2006, that was impossible to decide, since the now-defunct IFSA had contractually barred its athletes from competing in WSM. Savickas and Pudzianowski have competed against each other on several occasions in WSM competitions, though, so a comparison can still be made.

| 2002 | Pudzianowski, first; Savickas, second |
| 2003 | Pudzianowski, first; Savickas, second |
| 2004 | Savickas, second; Pudzianowski, third |
| 2009 | Savickas, first; Pudzianowski, second |

By the measuring stick of WSM competitions, it's a wash.

More telling is their head-to-head performance in another strongman contest—the Arnold Strongman Classic. From 2003 to 2005, Pudzianowski and Savickas competed against each other three times. Savickas, who competed in the ASC each year since 2003, had never lost the strongman contest [until 2010], although he took a year off in 2009. Pudzianowski came in fifth in 2003, fourth in 2004, and sixth in 2006. He did not compete in 2005, 2007, 2008, and 2009 although he was invited those years. Pudzianowski was not only dominated by the more massive Savickas in the ASC competitions, he was nothing more than mediocre in the process.

| 2003 | Savickas, first; Pudzianowski, fourth |
| 2004 | Savickas, first; Pudzianowski, fifth |
| 2006 | Savickas, first; Pudzianowski, sixth |

> Savickas, who competed in the ASC each year since 2003, had never lost the strongman contest [until 2010], though he took a year off in 2009.

Because of Savickas's dominance in his six ASCs and Pudzianowski's mediocre performance in each of his three ASC showings, many, I among them, think that Savickas, not Pudzianowski, is the real strongest man in the world.

Why has Pudzianowski tended to dominate WSM contests and been so mediocre in ASC?

### Types of contests

The reason concerns the types of events included in ASC and the manner in which they are contested. As I have argued in prior publications, WSM is a poor test for the strongest man in the world.[1] Overall, there are too many events—and there is always a qualifying round just prior to the actual contest; and the events contested are not customarily suitable tests of strength for a strongest man in the world contest. In contrast, the events contested in ASC are set up with the primary aim of being the best test for a strongest man in the world contest. The events are few and simple, and involve pushing, pulling, or overcoming massive weights.

Overall, I have argued that three criteria ought to be used in structuring a contest to determine who the strongest man in the world is: completeness, heaviness, and simplicity (CHS) criteria.

- Completeness: the contest should only include events that are complete, full-body (and not frivolous) tests of strength
- Heaviness: the contest should use weights that test the very limits of human strength
- Simplicity: the contest should include events that are relatively uncomplicated

Pudzianowski tends to do well in all WSM events, but many WSM contests have historically violated the CHS criteria. Pudzianowski excels in moving events, like the power stairs, the loading race, the car walk, the medley, the farmer's walk, and the shield carry. None of those events, however, are in keeping with the CHS criteria.

> IN CONTRAST, THE EVENTS IN WHICH SAVICKAS EXCELS—OVERHEAD PRESSING, SQUATTING, DEADLIFTING—ARE EVENTS THAT FIT WELL WITHIN THE CHS CRITERIA.

In contrast, the events in which Savickas excels—overhead pressing, squatting, deadlifting—are events that fit well within the CHS criteria.

There is, of course, more to say about my justification for the CHS criteria, but that is a subject for another article.

If we follow the CHS criteria, it is clear that Savickas, not Pudzianowski, is the true strongest man in the world. Moreover, Savickas, because of some of the records he has set and continues to set along the way, can justifiably claim to be the strongest person who has ever lived. M

---

[1] M. Andrew Holowchak, "What It Really Takes to be the World's Strongest Man: A Philosophical Investigation of Strength," *Philosophical Reflections on Physical Strength: Does a Strong Mind Need a Strong Body?* (New York: The Edwin Mellen Press, 2010) and "Testing for the World's Strongest Man," *Iron Game History* (forthcoming).

# Philosophy on Strength:

## What Makes a Person the Strongest?

**Paul Mouser**

Ongoing debates about what contest or method is the best at determining the strongest man in the world (the focus here is on men's competitions) populate message boards, weight shacks, and living rooms alike. The argument generally boils down to the World's Strongest Man (WSM) contest versus the Arnold Classic Strongman (ACS) contest. A third contest called Fortissimus emerged in 2008 and was held again in 2009, but the future of that show is uncertain at best, so it will not be discussed here. A strongman organization called IFSA also held a world championships, but it has since folded as well. Thus, the Arnold and the WSM will be the events that are examined in an effort to discover the best ways to determine strength.

The Arnold features six events over two days, and focuses on what are called "brute strength" events. The events are designed to minimize movement of the feet and to be extremely heavy, and thus limit the number of repetitions the competitors are able to perform to almost always single digits. The events generally contested at the Arnold (they change only slightly year to year) are:

1. Timber Carry – 875 lb. carried up a 36' ramp
2. Apollon's Wheels – 366 lb. on a non-revolving thick bar cleaned or continentaled and pressed or jerked for reps in 2 minutes
3. Tire Deadlift – a partial deadlift for maximum weight
4. Manhood Stones – super heavy spheres lifted over a bar for reps
5. Circus Dumbbell – 202-lb. thick-handled dumbbell pressed over head for reps
6. Super Yoke – 1100 lb. carried on the shoulders for 36'

Many would argue that these types of events are the proper way to determine strength, and they have some good arguments. The Arnold has been called the heaviest strongman contest ever by a guy who would know—strength historian David Webster, OBE. Mr. Webster also stated at the 2008 Arnold that the winner of the Arnold was truly the strongest man in the world.[1] The legendary Bill Kazmaier has stated that strength is best tested with minimal movement of the feet, and the Arnold showcases events that require movement of no more than 10 meters.[2] In fact, four of the six events require no movement of the feet at all. It seems hard to argue with Webster and Kaz, but a look at the World's Strongest Man contest may provoke more than a few protests against their ideas.

The World's Strongest Man contest differs from the Arnold in a host of ways: the show is contested over two weeks; there are seven events in the final alone, in addition to the six in the qualifiers; some of the events require movement of the feet until the competitor can move no longer; and some events call for repeated short sprints between implements. The point here is to both make good TV and to test different aspects of strength. The events from the 2008 World's Strongest Man final (I chose the 2008 show because I watched it live) were:

1. Power Stairs – a 500-lb. block with a handle carried up 20 stairs
2. Car Walk – 902 lb. carried on the shoulders over 90'
3. Fingal's Fingers – 5 poles of increasing weight (from 440 to 705 lb.) flipped over a pivot
4. Car Deadlift – 750 lb. deadlifted for reps in 75 seconds
5. Log Lift – 309 lb. cleaned or continentaled and pressed or jerked over head for reps
6. Plane Pull – a 40-ton plane pulled with a harness and rope over 90'
7. Atlas Stones – five stones increasing in weight from 220 to 400 lb. (the final stone was announced as 400 lb. in 2008, though in 2009 it was listed as 360 lb.) and lifted onto platforms of decreasing height starting from over 72" to about 54"

What makes the winner of these events a claimant to the title of World's Strongest Man? First, there are more events (remember there is a one-week qualifier), thus testing more aspects of strength. Second, many of these events focus on a type of strength that nearly everyone in the Iron Game has written about, functional strength. The Fingal's Fingers and the Barrel Loading (not listed here, since it was from the qualifier), for example, test strength in a way that barbells simply never could. Remember that four of the six events at the Arnold have handles to grab onto, whereas only three out of seven events at the WSM afford the men that luxury (the Plane is Pull is arguable, but I do not consider a rope a true handle, as it is awkward and pliable). The authors who have written about functional strength are too numerous to mention, but I must say that those who hold functional strength above all other types of strength are supporting the World's Strongest Man contest as the true determinant of the strongest man, intentionally or not.

So, which contest takes the cake? Here is the final rundown of the arguments for each contest.

### Arnold Strongman Challenge
- it's heavier—period
- limited movement involved, thus reducing agility and endurance factors
- TV production is not a factor in determining events
- contested over a shorter period, thus favoring the athlete who can best peak his strength

### World's Strongest Man
- more awkward, functional events
- more events in total
- contested over two weeks, thus favoring the athlete who can call upon his strength repeatedly
- tests more aspects of strength

We've discussed the contests, so now let's talk about the contestants. Two of the strongest men of our time, who just so happen to be fellow West Virginians, are Brian Siders and Phil Pfister. Brian and Phil are friends and have trained extensively together. They are, however, very different in their abilities and strengths. Mr. Siders is quite possibly the greatest powerlifter of all time. He totaled 2,601.5 lb. (a world record) in the gold standard organization of powerlifting, the IPF (by way of the affiliate USAPL).[3,4] He excels at the

Phil Pfister won the 2006 World's Strongest Man contest—the first American since Bill Kazmaier to reach this pinnacle of the strongman world. The low-key Phil Pfister's raw talent for strongman is staggering, so even though he's never been accused of overtraining or overachieving, winning the World's Strongest Man contest simply seemed a matter of fulfilling his destiny for the independent-thinking, sushi-eating strongman.

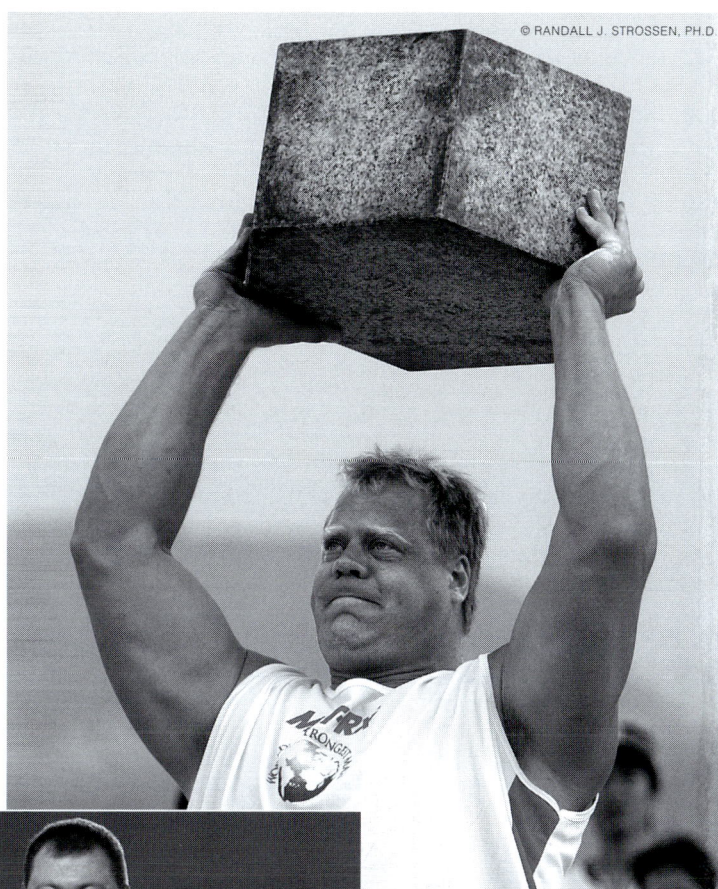

Brian Siders is a proven IPF powerhouse and even though he rarely competes in strongman, on selected events his tremendous strength is evident.

All photos by Randall J. Strossen.

Arnold Classic and, though he hasn't won the event yet, he did place ahead of Phil in 2008 and ran neck and neck with him for points in 2009. In the static events, like the Apollon's Wheels and the Tire Deadlift, Brian places consistently well and usually ahead of Mr. Pfister. Perhaps by Kazmaier's definition, Brian's powerlifting prowess alone could make him the strongest man in the world. Combine that with his success at the static strongman events and you have a guy that could very well be the true modern Samson.

Phil also does well at the Arnold, with his strengths being the Manhood Stones and the Circus Dumbbell—the more unwieldy of events. The contest where Phil truly shines, though, is of course the World's Strongest Man. Phil has placed fourth on three occasions and won the title in 2006. When both Brian and Phil competed in 2008, Phil made the finals and placed fourth, while Brian struggled in his qualifying group and missed the finals by a fair margin. Of particular difficulty for Brian was the Fingal's Fingers. Despite his unquestionable pressing, hip, and leg strength, Brian couldn't transfer his tremendous power to the Fingers. Phil has held the world record on the Fingers and the Atlas Stones, however, and thus from the functional strength perspective, his title of World's Strongest Man is undeniably legitimate. One must speculate that since Phil's most troublesome events are the squat and deadlift, should the two titans meet on the powerlifting platform, the roles would be reversed, with Brian setting records and Phil watching the competition pass him by.

So what does all of this tell us? For starters, Brian and Phil are both world-class athletes and two of the strongest men ever to live. Second, since Zydrunas Savickas is the only man to win WSM and the Arnold (as well as the IFSA Worlds and Fortissimus), he is currently the strongest man on Earth by almost anyone's definition. Aside from that, it comes down to preference and your personal philosophy: static strength versus functional strength.

Are these aspects mutually exclusive to one contest or the other? Of course not. Both shows have aspects of static and functional strength—each simply has an emphasis in one area more than the other. Certainly the people behind the contests could borrow from each other to continue to broaden their already fantastic shows. Adding a stone carry and/or barrel loading event (unwieldy events without handles) to the Arnold would likely please the functional strength crowd. Conversely, adding weight to the Atlas Stones and deadlift events (which many athletes finish now with strength to spare) at WSM would draw praise from the brute strength aficionados.

In the end, it is not about pleasing everyone, as such is the quest of fools; it is about finding the best ways to determine strength. Both shows have done so quite well to this point, and even with any possible changes, the debate, I imagine, will continue. M

Works cited:
1. GMV Productions. 2008 Arnold Strongman Classic [DVD]. 2008. Australia (2008).
2. IMG Sports Media. *Thirty Years of Pain: History of the World's Strongest Man* [DVD]. England (2006).
3. Men's Superheavyweight Weight Class Top 20. Soong, M. Retrieved on January 31, 2010 from http://www.powerliftingwatch.com/records/shw-men.
4. Men's American Records. Last updated on January 29, 2010. Retrieved on January 31, 2010 from http://www.goheavy.net/records/.

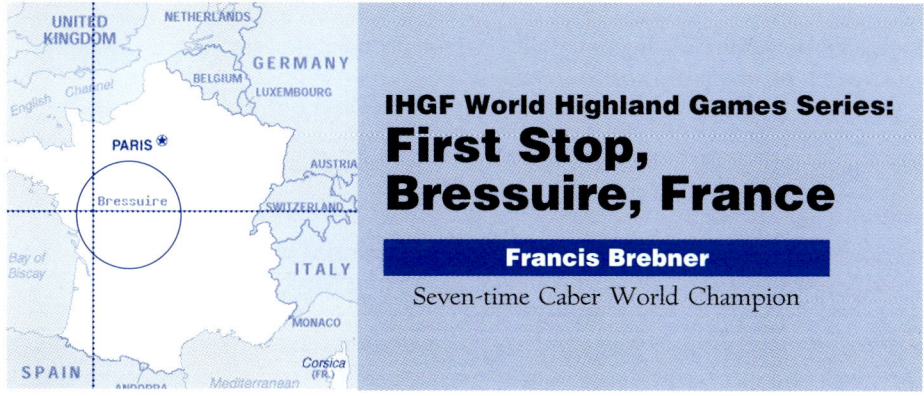

## IHGF World Highland Games Series: First Stop, Bressuire, France

### Francis Brebner
Seven-time Caber World Champion

The idea for a World Highland Games Super Series had been conceived several years ago and the first event had finally come to pass in Bressuire, France.

After a long journey from Los Angeles to Bressuire, I was happy to be staying with my wonderful host family, John and Corine Roy and their son Vincent, who is a great guitarist. On the Saturday morning of the Bressuire Games I awoke early to the ancient sound of the pipes as they echoed through the small forest. I looked out the window through the trees and I could see the castle as the sound beckoned, come, listen, come here, come compete.

The first day of the IHGF World Highland Games Super Series in Bressuire attracted big crowds who traveled from all over to get a glimpse of nine of the world's best heavy athletes doing battle at one of Europe's top Highland Games venues, the grounds of the thousand-year-old Bressuire Castle.

Jean-Louis Coppet and his committee did a remarkable job organizing every aspect of the Games, from the pipe bands to the dancing and folk music, making a winning formula for a successful traditional Games.

In the 22-lb. hammer, Betz won by showing great timing and speed, ripping out a distance of 113' 2". In second place was Larry Brock (USA) with 109' 7-3/4" and in third place was Scotland's Craig Sinclair with 108', which was not too bad considering that he had to throw without any boot spikes as his luggage got lost in transit from Scotland.

Next came the 17-lb. open stone, and it was very exciting as Rider obliterated the previous ground record held by Gregor Edmunds (Scotland) by nearly a meter and a half with a put of 57' 4-3/4". In second place was Betz with 51' 6-1/2", and in third place was Holland's Hans Lolkema with 51' 4-3/4".

The crowds were entertained in the 56-lb. weight for distance by another record-breaking performance as Brock sent the weight flying a incredible 46' 9-3/4", surpassing the previous ground record held by Lolkema by 3 m. Betz was in second place with 43' 7-3/4" and Rider in third place with a personal best of 42' 10-1/2".

The caber toss was the final event, and the caber, measuring a whopping 19 ft. and 150 lb., proved a real challenge and only three athletes were able to successfully toss this brute. Rider had the winning toss of 12:05; in second place was Brock with 9:30, and in third was Lolkema with 12:20.

After day one, Betz was in first with 9.5 points, Rider in second with 10, and Brock in third with 12.

On the second day of the Super Series, more records fell, including the size of the crowds. This year there were over 12,000 spectators flowing through the gates, which surpassed last year's record attendance of 10,000.

In the 16-lb. hammer there was a hard-fought skirmish between Brock, Sinclair, and Betz, with all three smashing Sinclair's previous ground record of 132'. Brock was the victor with a throw of 138' 6-1/2", with Sinclair in a very close second with 137' 10-1/4", and Betz in third with 136' 5".

The 22-lb. Braemar stone was next and it was also the final leg of the IHGF World Stone Putting Championships. The second record of the morning fell with both Rider and Betz overreaching the previous record held by Gregor Edmunds of 39' 5". Rider put 40' 3-1/4" for the win, with Betz coming in second with 39' 6-3/4" and Australia's Aaron Neighbour taking third with 37' 10-1/2".

In the 28-lb. weight for distance, the remaining ground record held by Gregor Edmunds of 81' 1" bit the dust big time as both Brock and Betz sent the weight flying over 85'. Brock landed a throw of 85' 10-3/4" for the win;

Betz came in second with 85' 3-1/2"; and Rider came in third with 80' 9-1/2".

The final record to crumble was the 56-lb. weight over the bar, formerly held by Wout Zjilstra of Holland at a height of 16' 5". There was no stopping Betz—he was on fire and feeding off of the thousands of spectators who were cheering him on—and he established the new record height of 16' 6", generating much applause from his many newfound fans. There was a tie for second place between Brock and Neighbour at 16' 1".

Overall winner Betz said, "I'm very happy with my throwing, it just all came together. As for Bressuire, without a doubt this has been the best experience competing around the world, number one for sure. I can't wait to compete here again. Jean-Louis Coppet and his amazing committee have done an awesome job with the Bressuire Games."

Rider came in second in the overall competition and first in the 2010 World Stone Putting Championships, followed by Betz and Neighbour.

**Overall points:**

| | |
|---|---|
| 1. Sean Betz (USA) | 17.5 |
| 2. Scott Rider (England) | 24 |
| 3. Larry Brock (USA) | 25 |
| 4. Aaron Neighbour (Australia) | 40 |
| 5. Ryan Vierra (USA) | 44.5 |
| 6. Greg Hadley (Canada) and Hans Lolkema (Holland) | 48.5 |
| 8. Craig Sinclair (Scotland) | 50 |
| 9. Petur Gudmunsson (Iceland) | 62 |

The next venue in the IHGF Super Series will be in Pleasanton, California, 4-5 September, and will include the 2010 World Caber and Weight-Over-Bar Championships.

## Cross Training:
# Bike Riding

**Steve Justa**

Author of *Rock Iron Steel: The Book of Strength*

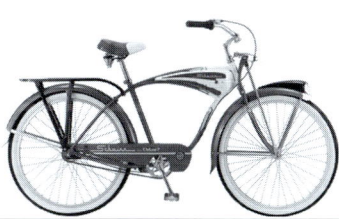

**B**icycle riding is a very good way to stay in shape on your off days between your heavy workouts. It is always fun to get out in the fresh air and get those lungs breathing good air—the air in some buildings, I must say, isn't the best quality.

I find when I ride my bike it is a very good way to get the poison out of my system and to keep the body running on all cylinders. All the food and water we drink nowadays seems to be contaminated with so many poisons and pollutants that it is very hard on the body—and going for a one- to two-hour bike ride is a very good way to work up a good sweat to clean the poison out of the system. I believe when you work up a good internal sweat, your body gets rid of a lot of these poisons through your sweat glands and in the long run keeps you more efficient.

> WHEN YOU'RE ON A BIKE YOU'LL SEE A LOT OF THINGS YOU JUST DON'T SEE WHEN YOU'RE IN A CAR.

You'll feel a whole lot better if you do something physical every day to get rid of that poison.

When I ride I usually go for a one- to two-hour ride. A two-hour ride for me usually translates into about 20 miles, and on a bike, this is about the right distance to get the job done.

When I ride I don't ride continually pedaling; I take my time and pedal a while and then coast, then pedal, then coast. I don't go in a straight line in town; I'll circle blocks and not be in a hurry to really get anywhere. I try to make the rides relaxing and fun—it is much more enjoyable that way and the time just flies by and before you even realize it, you've gone 20 miles.

When you're on a bike you'll see a lot of things you just don't see when you're in a car. It is a lot of fun to me and very relaxing and entertaining. I

> BIKE RIDING IS FOR ME VERY RELAXING AND A GOOD WAY
> TO KEEP MYSELF TUNED UP FOR THE HEAVY IRON.

like to watch the scenery and see what's going on. From time to time when I go downtown in a big city, I like to rest and just enjoy the scenery. I'll ride up alongside a building with a concrete step and stop and put one foot down and just rest a while, watching the traffic, and then I'll start up again. This is a very relaxing way to train and get the blood circulating.

What kind of bike you ride doesn't really matter just so you like it and it fits you comfortably. I would recommend you get those tires or tubes that are thorn-resistant—they are thicker and will save you a lot of hassle. It is not fun to get a flat tire on a bicycle if you don't carry the right tools to fix it. I would recommend that you go out and get the right wrenches that you can take your tires off with and also get one of those hand air pumps. Having the right tools will save you a lot of headaches, especially if you are riding out on the highway and are going to another town road-tripping and you break down and don't have anybody to call to help you or to come pick you up. I would also recommend that you carry some water with you and two or three of those energy bars, especially if you are going a long distance.

Bike riding is for me very relaxing and a good way to keep myself tuned up for the heavy iron. I would suggest you just ride as long as you want—don't put a time limit on it. It's great for your cardiovascular system. It'll take your body about a month or two to adjust to the extra work load, and it will probably drain your strength a little on the heavy lifts, so don't get frustrated. Be patient and your strength will come back and you'll be in better shape and start making really good progress. After a couple of months it will be easy for you to do 20 miles.

Bike riding is a lot of fun and I highly recommend it for everyone to really stay in better shape. It will pay off for you in the long run so go grab a bike and have some fun. **M**

> IT IS NOT
> FUN TO GET
> A FLAT TIRE
> ON A BICYCLE
> IF YOU DON'T
> CARRY THE
> RIGHT TOOLS
> TO FIX IT.

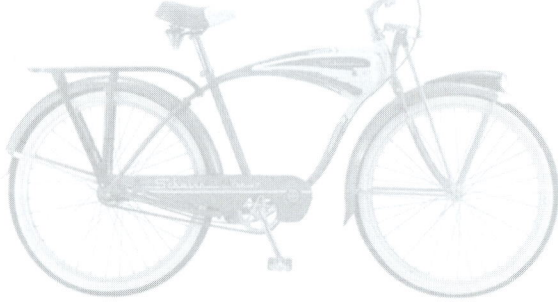

# The Iron Mine

## Websites, Training Forums

**Whelan Strength Training—20 Years!**
Olde-time physical culture studio in Washington, DC, building physically superior athletes and serious non-athletes. WhelanStrengthTraining.com. Phone consultation—WhelanStrengthTraining.net.

**Sustain Strength & Speed**
Battling Ropes: you read about them in *MILO*. Learn more about John Brookfield's strength and conditioning system at www.battlingropes.com.

**Strong and Healthy Hands for Everyone**
www.strongandhealthyhands.com.

**Join the IronMind Forum!**
If you love strength, the IronMind Forum is the place for you. We welcome all—experienced forum goers, newcomers and those in between. Join the fun. www.ironmind-forum.com.

**Captains of Crush Grippers Fans**
The facts, fiction, myths about Captains of Crush Grippers, and more: training programs, history highlights, gripper glossary, how-tos & FAQs—it's all here. www.captainsofcrushgrippers.com.

**PrimordialStrengthSystems.com**
Creating the most explosive athletes through the science of persistence.

**The IronMind News**
The Strength World's News Source. Fast. Accurate. Objective. www.ironmind.com.

**Follow IronMind on Twitter**
Twitter lets you stay in touch with us and receive up-to-the-minute blasts on the latest IronMind News and flashes from the field at major events.

## Equipment

**Real Wood Strongman Logs**
Slater's True Logs are built to last, used in top pro strongman contests. E-mail steve@slatershardware.com, 740-654-2204; www.slatershardware.com.

**Adjustable Grippers**
and strength training equipment. www.gripempire.com.

## Equipment

**World-class VULKAN Supports**
Heavy-duty, high-quality: knee, arm, back, & pants for strongman, powerlifters, heavy events, bodybuilders. Retail & wholesale. www.theweakgeteaten.com.

**Strongman Equipment**
Pulling harnesses, Slater's Stone Molds, True Logs, & Monster DBs, kettlebells, books, DVDs and more. www.totalperformancesports.com. 617-387-5998.

**Atlas Stone Molds from Slater's!**
Easy to make, hard to break, heavy-duty poly-Lexan, for time-after-time uses in 8, 10, 12, 14, 16, 18, 20, & 24-inch dia. Low int'l & dom. S&H. 740-654-2204. E-mail steve@slatershardware.com; dealers: www.slatershardware.com, www.totalperformancesports.com, www.marunde-muscle.com, www.prowriststraps.com.

**Strong, Pain-Free Hands**
In one convenient package: **three** vital training tools and guide for preventing, reducing, or eliminating hand pain. Kit includes IronMind EGG, Expand-Your-Hand Bands, Wrist-Relief Soft Weight, and booklet "How to Develop Strong, Pain-Free Hands." $51.85 + S&H: $13 USA, US$19 Canada, US$40 all others. Available in our on-line store at www.ironmind.com, or send payment to IronMind Enterprises, Inc., P.O. Box 1228, Nevada City, CA 95959 USA.

**IronMind Goods in Germany!**
Books, gear, equipment and MORE! www.c-of-c.de, Choice of Champions, Dr. Hermann Korte, Recklinghaeuser Str. 119, 45721 Haltern am See, Germany; e-mail info@k3k.de.

**Vulcan Racks Squat Racks**
Strong, simple, versatile, mobile, essential and at home in backyards, garages and gyms around the world. Just in case you, too, squat over 1,000 pounds, know that these racks are Shane Hamman strong, yet they are light enough to move around easily, and they break down in seconds for storage or workouts on the run. Available in our e-store at www.ironmind.com.

## Equipment

**Strength Equipment**
from the FIRST to close the No. 3 Captains of Crush Gripper. Custom super-duty racks, benches and selectorized machines by Sorinex. Owned, designed and tested to be virtually bombproof by Richard Sorin. 20+ years of experience supplying universities, gyms and serious lifters nationwide. Call and talk with The Grip Man at 877-767-4639, P.O. Box 121, Irmo, SC 29063; visit our websites at www.sorinex.com and www.sorinexforums.com

**Free Catalog: IronMind Enterprises Tools of the Trade for Serious Strength Athletes**
IronMind is the home of Captains of Crush® Grippers, *SUPER SQUATS*, Just Protein®, *MILO*®, the Vulcan Racks II+ System Squat Racks, Strong-Enough Lifting Straps™, and the Draft Horse Pulling Harness™, not to mention the world's leading line of grip tools, a top-quality line of gym equipment, strongman training equipment for the world's strongest men, and books, posters, and DVDs to inform and inspire you to greater success. While we sell plenty of equipment to champion strength athletes around the world, our specialty is the dedicated home trainer—strong guys who train in their garages, basements and backyards. Come take a look at what we have to offer. P.O. Box 1228, Nevada City, CA 95959 USA; t - 530-272-3579; f – 530-272-3095; website and on-line store: www.ironmind.com; e-mail: sales@ironmind.com.

## Associations

**The Association of Oldetime Barbell & Strongmen**
A not-to-be-missed annual reunion and dinner—this year, it's on October 23, 2010—for some of the biggest names in the Iron Game. Members receive a very interesting newsletter. Annual donation is $25, payable to AOBS, c/o Artie Drechsler, President, 33-30 – 150 Street, Flushing, NY 11354; email: lifttech@earthlink.net; www.wlinfo.com.

# The Iron Mine

## Associations

**Join USA Weightlifting!**
The National Governing Body for the Olympic sport. Go to www.usaweightlifting.org or call 719-866-4508, for news about recent competitions and courses, membership information, local and national events, coaching education, and the newest items available on-line. Membership benefits include participant accident insurance, a subscription to *Weightlifting, USA*, and **super discounts** on airline tickets, hotels, car rentals, and other products and services through our Olympic partnership!

## Training: Magazines, Books, DVDs

**Free Illustrated Catalog!**
Books, courses, back-date magazines, out-of-prints, new, etc. Classic how-to training methods and biographies by all the old masters. Buy, sell, trade, collecting over 40 years. Bill Hinbern, 32430-E Cloverdale, Farmington, MI 48336; www.superstrengthbooks.com.

*Powerlifting USA*
Contest results, schedules, training. 12 iss/year; $36.95 US; $96.00 elsewhere. PLUSA, P. O. Box 467, Camarillo, CA 93011; 800-448-7693.

*Real Strength Real Muscle*
This article anthology by the late Coach John Christy is for Real People with Real Lives: those who want to get bigger, stronger, and better conditioned without sacrificing family, school, or work. Real routines, real trainees, real answers, real nutritional guidance. 408 pp. $46.50 ppd. USA / US$71.50 ppd. others. DVDs also available. Order from www.realstrength-realmuscle.com/book.htm.

*Defying Gravity*
by Bill Starr. Signed. Hard cover $20, soft cover $15 + $5.00 S&H. Bill Starr, 1011 Warwick Drive, #3-C, Aberdeen, MD 21001.

**Starr Novel**
The Susquehanna River Hills Chronicles, a novel by Bill Starr. $20 + $6 S&H USA; 1011 Warwick Drive, #3-C, Aberdeen, MD 21001.

## Training: Magazines, Books, DVDs

**"The Steel Tip Newsletter"**
by Dr. Ken is once again available. www.oldtimestrongman.com. 1-800-978-0206.

*World Weightlifting*
The official magazine of the International Weightlifting Federation; its four issues a year cover contests worldwide. $40/year Europe, $50 elsewhere. World Weightlifting, IWF Secretariat, 1146 Budapest, Istvanmezei ut 1-3, Hungary.

*Bodyweight Exercises*
*For Extraordinary Strength:* if you follow Brad Johnson's advice, you will get very strong in a multitude of directions, and when it comes time to move your body around, it will feel like a feather. We won't guarantee that you'll be able to master the one-arm chin like Brad Johnson, but armed with this book, you can exceed your current best by a country mile. 72 pp. $13.95 plus S&H: $5/US; $7/Can; $13/all others; www.ironmind.com.

**The Get-Big-and-Strong Program**
*SUPER SQUATS: How to Gain 30 Pounds of Muscle in 6 Weeks*: This is the program that has turned human toothpicks into stalwarts and stalwarts into legends. After a few minutes under a squat bar, you will find out what you're made of; and if you want to get bigger and stronger and have no use for drugs, fancy equipment, or the latest food supplement fad, this is your book. 112 pp. $16.95 plus S&H: $5/US; $7/Can; $13/all others; www.ironmind.com.

**Denis Reno's Newsletter**
The quickest and best way to get Olympic weightlifting results, from local contests to World Championships. $26/year US, $30 Can., $45–$50 others. Denis Reno, 30 Cambria Road, Newton, MA 02165; e-mail: renoswlnl@verizon.net.

**Weightlifting Videos**
20 high-quality DVDs from every weight class of the 2006 USA W/L Nat. Jr. Champs & Pan-Am Qualifier, $30/session; e-mail WeightliftingVideoDirect@gmail.com for compressed samples or to order.

## Training: Magazines, Books, DVDs

**NEW! Battling Ropes DVD**
Featuring Ingrid Marcum, champion weightlifter and bobsledder this DVD shows you how to build strength and stamina using the unique Battling Ropes system developed by John Brookfield. Aimed at both individuals and teams, the system uses a long, heavy rope to train at high levels of intensity for longer durations, increasing your ability to generate and sustain power. Strongmen, football players, Special Forces types especially, you'll want this. 48 min., NTSC. $39.95 plus S&H: $5/US; $7/Can; $13/all others; www.ironmind.com.

**Updated! Captains of Crush Grippers book**
Whether you want to get an A+ on your next gripper exam or only care about building a stronger grip, you'll want to get this book—now updated and expanded to include over 45% new material, and most of it on training. Dedicated to all who know "it's not a crush . . . it's an obsession!" 192 pp. $19.95 + S&H: $5.00 USA, US$7.00 Can., US$13.00 all others. IronMind Enterprises, www.ironmind.com.

**Paul Anderson's Books and Tapes**
The Paul Anderson Youth Home offers a free catalog of Paul's books and tapes, as well as the Coleman video on Paul's life. This gives you a unique opportunity to learn from the world's strongest man while helping to support the youth home which Paul Anderson was dedicated to building. For a copy of this catalog, contact: Paul Anderson Youth Home, P. O. Box 525,

## The Iron Mine

Looking to buy or sell? Want to give your upcoming contest an extra boost? Advertise in the Iron Mine. $10 per line per insertion, no minimum number of lines. No display ads, please. All material subject to approval. Send advertising copy or direct questions to: *MILO*, P.O. Box 1228, Nevada City, CA 95959, tel 530-272-3579, fax 530-272-3095, sales@ironmind.com. *We try to screen the advertising, but let the buyer beware.*